# |WITHDRAWN|

# Clinical Perspectives on Elderly Sexuality

# Issues in the Practice of Psychology

SERIES EDITOR:

**George Stricker**, *Derner Institute of Advanced Psychological Studies,
Adelphi University, Garden City, New York*

---

CLINICAL PERSPECTIVES ON ELDERLY SEXUALITY
Jennifer L. Hillman

HANDBOOK OF QUALITY MANAGEMENT IN BEHAVIORAL HEALTH
Edited by George Stricker, Warwick G. Troy, and Sharon A. Shueman

PSYCHOTHERAPY AND BUDDHISM: Toward an Integration
Jeffrey B. Rubin

---

A Continuation Order Plan is available for this series. A continuation order will bring delivery of each new volume immediately upon publication. Volumes are billed only upon actual shipment. For further information please contact the publisher.

# Clinical Perspectives on Elderly Sexuality

## JENNIFER L. HILLMAN

*The Pennsylvania State University*
*Berks-Lehigh Valley College*
*Reading, Pennsylvania*

**KLUWER ACADEMIC/PLENUM PUBLISHERS**
NEW YORK, BOSTON, DORDRECHT, LONDON, MOSCOW

Library of Congress Cataloging-in-Publication Data

Hillman, Jennifer L.
    Clinical perspectives on elderly sexuality/Jennifer L. Hillman.
        p.   cm. — (Issues in the practice of psychology)
    Includes bibliographical references and index.
    ISBN 0-306-46335-0
        1. Aged—Sexual behavior.  2. Sexology—Research.  I. Title.  II. Series.

HQ30 .H55 2000
306.7′0846—dc21
                                                                        00-023541

ISBN: 0-306-46335-0

©2000 Kluwer Academic / Plenum Publishers, New York
233 Spring Street, New York, N.Y. 10013

http://www.wkap.nl/

10   9   8   7   6   5   4   3   2   1

A C.I.P. record for this book is available from the Library of Congress

Printed in the United States of America

To my family

# Preface

Throughout my clinical training and practice, I have been surprised by the number of times that sexual issues have emerged as an unexpectedly central feature in my work with older adults. I can vividly remember my own internal reaction on hearing one of my elderly female patients tell me that she was date raped a few years after the death of her elderly husband—when she was 68 years old. I can see in my mind's eye the blood splattered on the floor of an inpatient unit from an elderly man who smashed his arm through a window, furious that his antidepressant medication made it impossible to climax through masturbation. On a much less dramatic but equally important note, I think about the elderly amputee who told me softly about his fears of resuming sexual activity with his wife of 25 years. I also think about the elderly woman whose inability to take herself shopping to find fashionable, comfortable clothes to fit over her hunched shoulders and large breasts helped precipitate a serious depression. In sum, I learned early on that elderly sexuality is not just about how many times a week someone makes love. It is my hope that sharing these experiences and introducing the related theories, research, and interventions will assist other clinicians in dealing with these often challenging and clinically demanding situations.

Without my patients, this text would not have been possible. I continue to admire them for their ability to face various situations and challenges with dignity, honesty, creativity, and humor. Their willingness to share their experiences makes this book possible, and truly clinically relevant. This text also would not have been possible without the many outstanding professionals who supervised me in my early work, and my current colleagues and friends in research. These very important people include George Stricker, Michael Bibbo, Richard Zweig, Donna Chimera, Adrienne DeSimonne, Christine Li, Gregory Hinrichsen, Eileen Rosendahl, Patrick Ross, Thomas Skoloda, and Denise Hien.

I am forever indebted to my husband, Doug, and young son, Sean, for their love and patience during this endeavor. "Come grow old with me; The best is yet to be."

# Contents

# 1

# An Introduction to Elderly Sexuality

*Contrary to popular stereotypes, older adults as a group are more hetero-geneous than both young and middle aged adults. In recognition of this diversity, clinicians should only expect that the sexuality expressed among their elderly patients will be as unique and varied.*

## THE IMPORTANCE OF ELDERLY SEXUALITY

In prior decades, elderly sexuality has been viewed as having no real impor-tance, as a waste of professionals' time, or, at its worst, as an oxymoron. Only in recent years has elderly sexuality been addressed seriously and responsibly from a clinical, although not from a general societal, perspective. Empathic, attentive work from clinicians and researchers has allowed the field of elderly sexuality to gain increased respect as well as a measurable body of knowledge. With the change in our country's demographics, featuring a rapid increase in the sheer numbers of older people, and our society's greater tolerance for more open discussions of sexuality in general, it is only a matter of time before the substan-tial need for clinical expertise in elderly sexuality becomes readily apparent.

Older adults themselves represent a diverse population who may or may not engage in sexual behavior within the context of long-term marriage or more nontraditional relationships. They may engage in any variety of activities such as dating, cohabitation, affairs, same-sex relationships, abstinence, and mastur-bation, and they may have romantic relationships in community living, assisted living, or full nursing care facilities. Despite potential differences in physical health and living arrangements, elderly adults can and do engage in the same types of sexual behaviors as their younger counterparts, and like younger adults, they may be satisfied or dissatisfied with their sex lives. However, because older adults often face intense pressure from society to adopt a passive role, from adult children who influence the family dynamic to professional caregivers who may play a significant role in their day to day regimen, an understanding of the multidimensionality of elderly sexuality is essential.

## THE RELEVANCE OF THIS TEXT

This text is intended to provide up-to-date information and practical advice regarding clinical issues in elderly sexuality. Detailed case examples will be used throughout to illustrate both theoretical constructs and therapeutic techniques, thus providing a unique clinical perspective. Empirical research findings will be introduced in a clear, easy to understand manner, along with a critical assessment of the underlying research methodology. Although this book is geared primarily for mental health students and professionals (e.g., psychologists, psychiatrists, social workers, counselors, clergy), its material is quite suitable for physical therapists, occupational therapists, nutritionists, nurses, nursing home administrators, geriatricians, retirement home coordinators, and others who work with older adults. It also is important to note that the material within this volume would be of interest to an older adult who has questions about elderly sexuality, and to people of various ages who may be family members, loved ones, caregivers, or friends of such older adults.

This volume also is intended to be unique in that the topics covered represent many of the commonly neglected themes in elderly sexuality including: sensuality and sexuality with or without a partner; women's issues such as body image, breast cancer, and sexual abuse; men's issues such as impotence, prostate disease, and body image; sexuality within the context of disabilities such as Alzheimer's disease; legal and institutional issues; the impact of prescription and over-the-counter medications, cross-cultural perspectives; hetero- and homosexuality, and HIV and AIDS. This introductory chapter is designed to provide a general overview of elderly sexuality, featuring societal attitudes and stereotypes, historical approaches, and an introduction to research methodology. Chapters 2 and 3 introduce basic, requisite knowledge of elderly sexuality, as well as suggestions for therapists in establishing open communication with patients and coping with a variety of attitudes toward elderly sexuality, including transferences and countertransferences.

The next two chapters highlight elderly sexuality within an institutional context such as a nursing home (Chapter 4) and within the context of disabilities and chronic illness such as depression, diabetes, arthritis, and Alzheimer's disease (Chapter 5). Chapter 6 discusses the often ignored and overlooked topics of high-risk sexual behaviors, HIV, and HIV-induced dementia among older adults. Chapters 7 and 8 are respectively devoted to specific women's and men's issues in elderly sexuality. Chapter 9 covers both traditional and nontraditional relationships among older adults as they relate to sexuality, and Chapter 10 concludes with a "look to the future" of elderly sexuality. This final chapter is devoted to a review of the clinical issues that are likely to emerge among an aging cohort of baby boomers, suggestions for coping with the medicalization of elderly sexuality (e.g., how to work more effectively in interdisciplinary settings), and the overall, positive notion that holding knowledge of elderly sexuality is the key to providing effective clinical care to the increasing numbers of older adults in our country.

## THE DEMOGRAPHICS OF AGING

### Defining Older Adulthood

In order to discuss older adulthood as a developmental stage or specific age cohort, it is necessarily to first define the age at which one becomes an "older adult." A number of arguments can be made to support the notion that older adulthood is not a function of chronological age, but rather a function of physical ability and mental health. Many older adults who exercise, eat properly, maintain fulfilling personal relationships, or possess a variety of "good genes" are in better mental and physical health than their younger counterparts who have a more sedentary or isolated lifestyle. Other experts maintain that the wisdom accumulated through life provides older adults with protection from stressful life events, and that an increase in the exploration of opposite-sex roles generates a youthful outlook among many chronologically older adults (Gutmann, 1994). As people age, we ourselves tend to regard older adulthood as beginning at later and later ages. However, for the sake of analyzing demographics and making some generalizations, it becomes helpful to view a specific, yet somewhat arbitrary age as a cutoff point for older adulthood. For ease of categorization in this text, older and elderly adults will be defined as men and women who are 65 years of age or older.

Although 65 years of age has been accepted generally as a defining point for older adulthood, it also is readily apparent to epidemiologists that adults who range from 65 to well over 100 represent a diverse group. Society itself tends to view (i.e., stereotype) a 65-year-old quite differently than a 95-year-old (e.g., Hummert, Garstka, Shaner, & Strahm, 1995). Although age 65 has been defined historically as the requisite age of retirement by the Social Security Administration, this age of retirement is already slated to increase within the next decade and is likely to advance over time as more older adults work later into life for both financial reasons and personal satisfaction. Also, the current cohort of older adults over the age of 85 appears to represent a unique subgroup of older adults, and they have been labeled as the oldest-old. These oldest-old adults have been identified as a group of adults who may require additional clinical attention and consideration because of their advanced age (e.g., Hillman, Stricker, & Zweig, 1997) and greater likelihood of experiencing chronic illness, poverty, and lack of social support (e.g., Pennix, et al., 1999).

### Relevant Statistics

Despite the heterogeneity of the older adult population, one fact is clear, namely, this segment of our population is increasing at a relatively rapid rate. A number of sources (e.g., U.S. Bureau of the Census, 1993, 1996) indicate that in 1990, about 1 in 8, or 31.1 million Americans were over the age of 65. Between the years 1990 and 2020, the elderly population will increase to more than 54 million people, representing 1 of every 6 Americans. From 1990 to 2050, the elderly population is expected to double in size to more than 79 million people. Put another way, in 2050, 1 in 5, or *20%*, of all Americans will be over the age of 65. This growth rate among the elderly population is nearly double that of the growth rate of the country's total population. A lengthier life span, better access to better health care, and the large numbers of aging baby boomers contribute to this rapid population increase. For example, the first members of the baby boom generation will begin to celebrate their 65th birthdays in the year 2011.

The diversity of the elderly population also is increasing in terms of race and ethnicity, poverty status, education, numbers of men and women, and marital status. Between 1990 and 2050, the numbers of elderly African-Americans are expected to quadruple from 2 to more than 9 million people. In other words, from 1990 to 2050, the number of African-Americans who are elderly is expected to double from 8% to more than 15% of their population. Among American Indians and Eskimos, their proportion of elderly adults is expected to double from 6% to more than 12%. Among Hispanic and Asian-Americans, the ranks of their elderly members are expected to nearly triple from 6% to 16%, and 5% to 15%, respectively. The absolute number of Hispanic elderly people estimated to be living in 2050 (more than 12 million) will be 11 times the number of Hispanic elders living in 1990. Diversity among the elderly also is apparent in their distribution of income. Although significantly more elderly people live above the poverty line than in 1970, elderly women continue to have nearly double the chance of living in poverty than elderly men; 16% of elderly women versus only 8% of elderly men live below the poverty line. Elderly adults with higher rates of education also are more likely to have more disposable income and retirement savings. All of these demographic changes are relevant when considering issues of elderly sexuality.

Within the cohort of elderly people aged 65 and older, the oldest-old segment of the population (i.e., aged 85 years and older) demands special attention as a unique subgroup. This group of the oldest-old is experiencing an even higher rate of growth than their young-old peers. In 1990, 3 million Americans were more than 85 years of age, representing approximately 1.2% of the nation's total population. By the year 2050, the number of oldest-old Americans is expected to reach more than 18 million people—a sixfold increase in their population since 1990. Related more directly to elderly sexuality and other societal and clinical issues, striking differences exist between men and women who belong to this oldest-old cohort. For example, the vast majority of the oldest-old population is comprised of women. For those aged 85 to 89 years of age, there are more than 2.5 women for every man. Among people aged 95 years and older, women begin to outnumber men by 4 to 1. These ratios are even more striking when one considers the numbers of single or "available" elderly men and women. (This assumes that there are issues of supply and demand among heterosexual elders; it remains virtually unknown what proportion of elderly men and women consider themselves homosexual. Ostensibly, lack of an available homosexual partner would be more of an issue for elderly men than for elderly women.) By age 85, nearly 1 out of 2 men are married, whereas nearly 4 out of 5 women

(80%) are widowed. Although men are expected to live almost as long as their female counterparts during the next century, there will continue to be a dramatic shortage of elderly men compared to elderly women.

## INTIMACY, SEXUALITY, SENSUALITY

In any discussion of sexuality, the differences and similarities between human intimacy, sexuality, and sensuality must be reviewed. Because various researchers and theorists have defined these terms differently, the meanings ascribed to them here should be regarded as generalizations and aids in nomenclature rather than theoretically driven constructs. The following categorizations are offered for the following:

1. *Intimacy* can be defined as the quality of the interpersonal relationship among two people in a romantic relationship, who may or may not be actively engaged in sexual relations. Attachment style, prior family dynamics, sexual identity issues, and self-esteem may all contribute to the level of intimacy experienced (or desired) by an individual. In practical terms, intimacy could be manifested by a subjective feeling of love or satisfaction when in the partner's presence or when thinking about the partner, the degree of appropriate self-disclosure between partners, and the willingness or ability to value the partner's needs and desires as well as one's own. For the purposes of this text, *intimacy* will be used to refer exclusively to emotional intimacy (i.e., interpersonal satisfaction and subjective feelings of closeness).
2. *Sensuality* can be defined as the experience of pleasure from one's senses leading to an increased awareness of and appreciation for one's own body. Such pleasure may be generated via sexual activity specifically, but also from any activation of the sensory organs. It is essential to note that sensual pleasure can be experienced with or without another person, and that expressions of sensuality are vast and quite individualized. Examples of sensual activities may include taking a hot bath or shower, noticing the breeze against one's face, having a massage, listening to music, lighting candles, getting one's hair done, eating a wonderful meal, molding or shaping clay, dressing up in beautiful clothing, splashing in puddles, lying in a feather bed, wearing silky underwear, singing in a resonant choral group, holding hands, using fragrant body lotions, dancing, engaging in foreplay, feeling muscles warm and loosen during exercise, or appreciating artwork. While sensual activities may induce sexual excitement, the inherent goal of the activity is not sexual intercourse or climax.
3. *Sexuality* will be defined here as a *broadly based* term that indicates any combination of sexual behavior, sensual activity, emotional intimacy, or sense of sexual identity. Any individual's wish to engage in any of these activities also may be considered an aspect of sexuality. Sexuality may involve sexual activity with the explicit goal of achieving pleasure or

climax (e.g., kissing, foreplay, intercourse), sensual activity with or without the explicit goal of achieving sexual pleasure (e.g., wearing body lotion to feel attractive or feminine), or the experience of emotional intimacy within the context of a romantic relationship. Thus, sexuality incorporates a vast number of issues including body image, masturbation, love, libido, intercourse, homophobia, relationship satisfaction, marital satisfaction, desires for sexual and sensual experience, and participation in high-risk behaviors. It also is important to note that sexuality encompasses thoughts, feelings, and behaviors that may lead to positive *or* negative feelings (e.g., consider body image, masturbation, and sexual abuse).

## THE HISTORICAL CONTEXT

It is useful to view contemporary societal attitudes toward elderly sexuality through the lens of historical attitudes. Consistent with current, dismissive attitudes toward elderly sexuality, little has been recorded about elderly sexuality in the art or literature of biblical and medieval times. However, the overwhelming majority of these few reports are negative (e.g., Covey, 1989). During these periods in history, sexual relations among older people were viewed as evil, immoral, perverse, inappropriate, impossible, or pathetically comical, at best.

During the Middle Ages in Europe, the church played a central role in shaping beliefs about elderly sexuality. At the core of these beliefs was the prohibition that sexual intercourse was designed for procreation only, among people of all ages. St. Augustine wrote that celibacy was a human ideal to strive for, and St. Albertus Magnus and St. Thomas Aquinas professed similar views that sex was for reproductive purposes only. This doctrine promoted great hostility toward older adults who engaged in any type of sexual behavior, as they engaged in a "sin against nature" (Bullough, 1976).

These religious prohibitions also were mirrored by general beliefs among the populous that sexuality was reserved for younger adults who could reproduce and multiply. Older adults were seen as entering an "age of life" in which decay, decline, and repose were an inescapable and unavoidable part of life (Burrow, 1986), even by preeminent scholars and scientists. In his *Masterpiece*, Aristotle wrote that sexual activity ceased for women at menopause and for men after their fifth decade of life (Stone, 1977). Other medieval physiologists professed that women had a stronger sex drive than men, but believed that this powerful drive ceased immediately on menopause. Thus, sexual activity among older adults was viewed as unnatural, inappropriate, and even disgusting. Consistent with this view, religious notions held that if older adults engaged in physical intimacy, they literally chained themselves to the flesh and impeded their ascension into heaven (Burrow, 1986).

Despite strong prohibitions against elderly sexuality in the Middle Ages, facets of popular culture suggest that this phenomenon was present but hidden, as represented in plays and famous literature. Chaucer provided an account of elderly sexuality in his *Canterbury Tales*. In the "Merchant's Tale," he describes a 60-year-old knight who wants to marry a young bride in order to satiate his sexual appetite. The implication is that older women simply do not have the ability (or attractiveness) to satisfy a man's needs: "I'll have no woman 30 years of age. That's only fodder ... straw for a cage." Chaucer also prompts his older knight to blatantly disregard church prohibitions about elderly sexuality: "A man is not a sinner with his wife, he can not hurt himself with his own knife." However, on his wedding night, the noble drinks large quantities of an aphrodisiac and falls asleep without consummating the marriage. When he becomes blind a few years later, the knight's young bride has an affair with one of his young servants. In a cruel twist of fate, the older knight regains his eyesight to the sight of his bride and servant making love in a field. As a further insult, his young bride convinces the older knight that he was just imagining things, because surely he has become senile at his advanced age. Although designed to be humorous, this story illustrates medieval beliefs that older men are not virile, are not attractive to younger women, are physically ill, and appear foolish if they attempt to engage in sexual relations. The story's other implications are that all older women are inherently unattractive and unable to obtain partners for sexual enjoyment.

Sex Differences

Thus, it can be assumed that although older adults did indeed show interest and engage in sexual relations during biblical and medieval times, these practices were regarded as hapless, humorous, and even dangerous by the general population. A double standard prevailed regarding male and female elderly sexuality, namely, that men's participation in sexual activity was seen as humorous or as a foolish possibility, whereas older women's participation in sex was viewed as unnatural and evil (Covey, 1989). For example, although older men were thought to have virtually no capacity for sexual relations, those who were able to have active sex lives were believed to gain social status and even an increase in their life span. In contrast, an older woman was thought only to have sex in her later years if she were able to trick a man into going to bed with her, a feat so abhorrent that it required the aid of witchcraft. This evilness associated with female elderly sexuality persisted well into the fifteenth century, fueled by the *Hammer of Witches*, a popular text indicating that witchcraft was responsible for both carnal lust among older women (Stone, 1977) and impotence among older men (Bullough, 1976).

## CROSS-CULTURAL PERSPECTIVES

An appreciation of cross-cultural perspectives on elderly sexuality is essential for an understanding of our current societal perspectives. Unfortunately, few quantitative or qualitative accounts exist to detail attitudes and practices about elderly sexuality in other cultures. What little information we do have, however, presents a picture that is strikingly different from that espoused by our industrialized North American, youth-oriented culture. An ancient Turkish proverb illustrates the general positivity espoused by the majority of traditional and preindustrial cultures: "young love is from earth, while late love is from heaven."

In a groundbreaking study of more than 106 cultures (Winn & Newton, 1982), less than 3% of those cultures were found to have societal sanctions or prohibitions against older people having sex. An analysis of the data gathered by the anthropologists, sociologists, and psychologists studying these cultures revealed that 70% and more than 84% of the societies reported sexual activity among its older male and female members, respectively. In many Eastern and Middle Eastern cultures, men commonly engaged in sexual relations well beyond the age of 100 and 80, respectively. African cultures maintained that impotence was not a normal function of old age, but an unnatural loss of ability resulting from illness or witchcraft. In the majority of these traditional cultures, menopause was not associated with either more or less sexual activity among older women; it simply represented a "point in a woman's life." In certain African and Asiatic cultures, an older women's physical attractiveness appeared unrelated to her sexual status; toothless, older women were considered as sexually desirable as younger women. Thus, sexual activity among older men and women in traditional societies is common, and apparently readily accepted, throughout most of the world.

An additional difference noted between these traditional societies and our own was that although a double standard appeared to operate with regard to elderly sexuality, it appeared to be in the opposite direction. Specifically, older women were more likely to engage in sexual relations than older men, and older women were often described (in more than one-fourth of the cultures) as becoming less sexually inhibited and more sexually aggressive with age. In certain South American and Eastern cultures, older women were designated teachers for sexually inexperienced young men. Older women also were described as commonly taking younger men for husbands or sex partners, ostensibly because there were few male partners available of their own age. Other older women in South American, Eastern, and North American Indian cultures were described as dressing more seductively, baring their breasts more often in public, and delighting in off-color jokes once past the age of 60.

## SOCIETAL STEREOTYPES

### The Implied Value of Youth

In contrast to these generally accepting attitudes among other world cultures, our contemporary societal attitudes toward elderly sexuality are ageist and highly negative. Butler (1969) first coined the term *ageism* as treating elderly persons differently and negatively, based solely on their advanced age. Consistent with this notion, most segments of our society posit that while sexuality is an essential, desirable, enjoyable part of life, elderly sexuality either does not exist, or that it is dirty, disgusting, and taboo. This derision for elderly sexuality has been documented extensively among college students, adult children of elderly adults, health care providers, and even among some older adults themselves.

The crux of the problem appears to be that sexuality, as well as other perceived societal benefits, is thought to be reserved for the young. Our culture values youth extensively for it represents independence, excitement, physical prowess, physical attractiveness, and the potential for growth and change. The American Dream implies that a younger person can do better than his or her parent (or grandparent), and the capitalistic component of our society places incredible value on a person's ability to work, earn a living, and secure even greater independence and autonomy. Although most members of our society accept these values and champion a strong work ethic, the implications for older adults can be devastating. Older adults who may be retired, physically disabled, or who no longer fit traditional standards of physical beauty, much less the majority who function happily and well in the community, are saddled with preconceptions that they are a useless burden to others, and no longer entitled to societal benefits such as love and sex.

## The Paradox of Elderly Sexuality

Although pervasive stereotypes exist that older adults are helpless, depressed, and sexless, another force in our society is to maintain youth, or at least its illusion, at any cost. Thus, we see multimillion dollar industries based on cosmetics, plastic surgery, exercise equipment, vitamin supplements, and retirement planning. Older adults also are expected to follow suit and dismiss any positive aspect of aging (e.g., wisdom, generativity, and acceptance of one's body and appearance) in order to seek the proverbial fountain of youth. A paradox ensues in which older adults are expected to be hapless, helpless, asexual beings who simultaneously are expected to be physically fit, completely independent, and sexualized beings. Thus, older adults in our culture appear destined to fail; while society cannot accept that an older adult is sexually active, it continues to insist that sexual behavior in late life is a goal that must be achieved.

## THE OEDIPAL COMPLEX REVISITED

From a psychodynamic perspective, Freud's introduction of the oedipal complex contributes to our understanding of the pervasively negative attitudes toward elderly sexuality espoused in most industrialized, Western cultures. Essentially, the oedipal conflict emerges when a child falls in love and wants to have sex with his opposite-sex parent. The child also may experience a desire to kill off (and compete with) his same-sex parent. Because incest is taboo in our society, these urges must be repressed, and the child ultimately develops a revulsion toward the thought of sex with his opposite-sex parent in order to avoid this oedipal conflict. This guilt-induced revulsion becomes repressed further and translated into general revulsion at the thought of one's parents, as a couple, engaging in any sexual activity whatsoever. A distaste for elderly sexuality is believed to be just as powerful and guilt-ridden because it represents the adult child's continued, unconscious need to renounce any sexual activity even loosely associated with parental sexuality (Kernberg, 1991). Thus, the societal taboo against elderly sexuality is likely to begin at a very early age.

The oedipal conflict also can be framed in terms of Darwinian concepts. Darwin observed that in many groups of primates, an older dominant male chased off the younger males so that he could mate with the large number of females in his collective. Sometimes, the younger males worked together in a primal horde (Freud, 1913/1946) or independently to kill the older male so that they could spread their now superior genetic material. This Darwinian observation is mirrored in Freud's supposition that during the resolution of the oedipal conflict, young boys must come to terms with their competitive and aggressive feelings toward their governing fathers. To expand this metaphor further, current demographics suggest that there are many more older females available and few older males. It may be a natural Darwinian response for older males to take a protective stance, and for younger males (i.e., the younger generation) to ward off any sexual competitors. Rather than resorting to physical violence as in the animal kingdom, another approach is for younger adults to render older adults, through the belief system of their society, as asexual beings who are not capable of engaging in sexual activity. Thus, if popular culture views older adults as nonsexual beings, older adults begin to internalize these beliefs and they lose their abilities as sexual competitors (Covey, 1989; Pfeiffer, 1977). This process guarantees the younger cohort virtually unlimited access to all sexual partners and resources.

## ELDERLY SEXUALITY IN THE POPULAR MEDIA

Mirroring Freudian oedipal theory and its corollary that people experience significant anxiety in response to elderly sexuality, representations of elderly sexuality traditionally have been absent or negative in the popular media. Surveys of various entertainment media (e.g., books, theatrical productions, periodicals) show that elderly sexuality has been historically underrepresented throughout the 1970s, particularly in television. This relative dearth of older adults in the popular media has the potential to influence older adults' views of themselves, as older adults are among the age group that watches the most television (Bell, 1992). It thus can be quite informative to ask our older adult patients what they read and what they watch on television in order to help them evaluate their own lives in relation to the artificially generated images portrayed in print or on screen (e.g., Kaiser & Chandler, 1988).

## Unexpectedly Positive Portrayals

Findings from various research studies suggest that in print media, older adults frequently are portrayed as cognitively impaired, annoying, lonely, stubborn, depressed individuals whose lives revolve around loss and illness. Positive social interactions, much less positive expressions of sexuality, do not appear to play a role in their lives (e.g., Nussbaum & Robinson, 1984). In contrast, portrayals of older adults in prime time television programs appear to be somewhat more positive. Qualitative research findings suggest that older adults in these programs tend to be engaged in positive social interactions, particularly within the context of familial settings. They also have been shown, on average, to perform tasks that require some degree of social and interpersonal independence (Dail, 1988) and to be stereotyped or typecast as individuals who are healthy, wealthy, agentic, and sexy (Bell, 1992).

Unfortunately, these positive portrayals of sexy, powerful older adults on television are more likely to stem from strategic marketing campaigns designed to capture the growing older adult market (e.g., Schewe & Balazs, 1992) than from a generation of more positive societal stereotypes regarding older adults and their sexuality. These attempts by Hollywood executives and advertising executives to show older adults in a positive, attractive, healthy, and sexy manner often are targeted specifically at an aging generation of baby boomers, who command significant buying power and represent a recently ignored consumer product base. Thus, the outcome appears to be an increase in the use of physically attractive, older adult characters in the media who may engage in sexual activity.

## Underlying Motives and Stereotypes

One may question whether it really matters whether capitalistic or egalitarian forces are responsible for the increase in positive media imagery regarding elderly sexuality. This increase in positive representations would seem to be a good omen, regardless of its actual source. However, taking a more than cursory look at this increase in positive media portrayals reveals some subtle but pervasive stereotypes. First, older adults tend to be portrayed in only one specific way; if they are not healthy, wealthy, and sexy, they do not seem to exist on prime time television. This lack of diversity, which certainly is not representative of the heterogeneity of the older adult population, can impact very negatively on older adults (Nussbaum & Robinson, 1984) who may have health problems, live in relative financial distress, or feel dissatisfied with their own sex lives. Older adults may feel as though they are not able to live up to some unattainable standard, or that they simply cannot compete with the attractive actors selected to appear in these prime time shows and advertisements.

Second, the context in which elderly sexuality is portrayed on television is circumscribed, stereotypical, and gender biased (Bell, 1992). Although prime time shows employ physically attractive characters who may flirt with members of the opposite sex, they rarely if ever engage in actual sexual behavior (e.g., kissing, lounging in bed). The older male characters in many shows who gain admiring glances from women seem to gain favor only from younger women, not women from their own age cohort. These male protagonists also are depicted as more "safe" (i.e., gentle and romantic) than virile and sexually dynamic. No consistent love interests or male characters are present in the prime time shows that feature older women characters. It is as though older women on television exist contentedly in a chaste sexual vacuum. Thus, although elderly sexuality (via sexy older men) may appear on prime time television, its context is limited, stereotypical, and not representative of elderly sexuality within the general population.

## UNDERSTANDING RESEARCH METHODS

In any introduction to elderly sexuality, it also is important to address differences in clinical research methods. The use of a scientist-practitioner model has earned the field increased respect as well as a relatively large knowledge base. Despite this increased knowledge base, however, inherent problems exist in conducting and interpreting sexuality research, much less in conducting and interpreting elderly sexuality research. Clinicians who are informed about the differences between empirical research (including both quantitative and qualitative approaches) and case studies are better able to evaluate these methods' findings and to apply them to practice. Although these different research methods are all valuable in their own right, the findings from each must be judged according to their own strengths and weaknesses.

Empirical research often is regarded as the least clinical of all types of research. However, acknowledging the ability of this approach to track general norms or societal trends can provide essential information to guide clinical practice. For example, quantitative research findings regarding epidemiological estimates of older adults who have contracted HIV (including the finding that more than half of all new AIDS cases in Palm Beach County, Florida, are among adults over the age of 50) can be used to dispel established, ageist stereotypes. These empirical findings suggest that older adults are sexually active people who may engage in high risk behaviors such as intravenous drug use, sex with multiple partners or prostitutes, and homosexual and heterosexual anal sex. Thus, seemingly "sterile" quantitative research findings can be used to enable clinicians to feel more confident and justified in their willingness to conduct a thorough clinical interview.

Unfortunately, such empirical research findings can also be highly influenced or biased by differences in subject sampling, instrument selection, and self-report biases. One major problem with empirical research is that one finding cannot necessarily be generalized to all members of this heterogeneous population. Regarding a likely increase in the occurrence of eating disorders among elderly women (Hsu & Zimmer, 1988), it becomes important not to generalize these findings to women of color. Because the vast majority of these studies have employed white subjects, and because African-American women have been shown to have greater satisfaction with their bodies (Hebl & Heatherton, 1998), it remains unclear whether elderly African-American women, as compared to their white counterparts, would be as likely to manifest eating disorders in later life. These limitations in subject sampling often lead to problems in over-generalizing research findings. In other words, if not interpreted properly, empirical research findings can be misconstrued and promote inappropriate stereotypes themselves.

The use of instrument or measurement selection in empirical research also can be problematic. If a test for knowledge of elderly sexuality has only true and false items, and the older adults in the study demonstrate little knowledge of elderly sexuality as revealed by a low average score, it remains unclear whether the older adults who took this test were generally unaware of the physiology of elderly sexuality. It also is possible that the participants were unable to understand the medical terms selected by the researcher, irritated that the test was so long, which led them to stop answering items carefully after approximately half an hour, unable to read the test items because the experimenter failed to remind them to bring reading glasses, or offended at questions regarding masturbation and homosexuality because of their religious beliefs, which led them to answer the remaining questions randomly. When asked to respond to self-report items, individuals also are more likely to under- and overestimate their participation in sexual behaviors (Bradburn & Sudman, 1979), perhaps in response to religious, societal, and cultural demands including ideals of purity and machismo (Catania, Gibson, Chitwood, & Coates, 1990).

In contrast to such quantitative research, which typically relies on printed, forced-choice measures, the use of qualitative research is more likely to employ open-ended questions and one-on-one subject interviews. This qualitative approach has become more common in elderly sexuality research because it generally allows for greater exploration of individual subjects' thoughts, feelings, and motivation. However, the use of such open-ended questions also relies on experimenter skill, consistency and training among interviewers, increased time requirements for both experimenters and participants, and the need for complicated statistical procedures to code and analyze the data. The use of qualitative approaches also presents its own unique problems and challenges. The age and sex of the interviewer can influence the results (i.e., gay men appear more likely to discuss their sexual activities with male than female interviewers), as can the actual mode of data collection. For example, study participants are more likely to admit that they engage in specific sexual behaviors if they are interviewed over the telephone than in person (Catania et al., 1990). Issues of privacy, concerns about self-presentation, and subject motivation (e.g., what can we infer about someone who is willing to volunteer a couple of hours to participate in a study about sexuality?) also appear heightened in these qualitative study formats.

Another important means of gathering information about elderly sexuality is through the use of case studies. The case also appears most closely aligned with traditional clinical practice, and allows for an in-depth understanding and appreciation for one patient's experience. All aspects of the individual involved are reviewed and discussed, including personal history, interpersonal relationships, cultural background, religious views, family dynamics, socioeconomic status, internalized beliefs and values, ethnic background, treatment progress, object relations, cognitive schemas, and any other relevant information. Although averages derived from quantitative research do provide critical information and can dispel unrealistic stereotypes, they inherently ignore individuals' unique histories and personal situations. The use of a case study also allows clinicians to recognize similarities and differences in their own approach to a patient's problem, and to gain exposure to sometimes obscure or previously unencountered clinical issues. In contrast, clinicians also must differentiate between case studies and clinical anecdotes. While interesting and often illuminating, clinical anecdotes represent only a fragment of a patient's (and practitioner's) experience, and must be viewed with the appropriate, critical stance.

## A BRIEF REVIEW OF THE LITERATURE

A brief overview of the literature on elderly sexuality suggests that we should not ascribe to societal stereotypes that older adults are helpless, passive, asexual beings not entitled to companionship, love, or sex. A number of researchers are quick to point out that many elderly men engage in sexual intercourse well into their 80s and 90s (Call, Sprecher, & Schwartz, 1995; Starr & Weiner, 1981), that elderly women tend to continue to enjoy satisfying sexual relations in their later years if they enjoyed satisfying sexual relations in their younger years (Janus & Janus, 1993; Matthais, Lubben, Atchison, & Schweitzer, 1997), and that the vast majority of older adults are healthy, community living members of society. In contrast to these glowing findings, other research findings suggest that impotence is the most common cause of sexual dysfunction and dissatisfaction among older men (Cogen & Steinman, 1990; National Institutes of Health, 1993) and that up to one-third of older women experience pain during intercourse and do not understand why or how to treat it (Bachmann, 1995; Jones, 1994). Older adults also are more likely to experience sexual dysfunction as a result of adverse drug reactions, as compared with young and middle-aged adults, and older adults, who represent only 13% of the general population, account for approximately 33% of all over-the-counter and prescription drug use (Dorgan, 1995).

In some cases, the absence of information in the literature is just as notable as the presence of other information. Most strikingly, virtually no research exists regarding the sexuality of *minority elders, gay and lesbian older adults, older adults living with disabilities, and the oldest-old members* of our society. This absence of attention to these populations in the literature may reflect a general societal disavowal of these groups that has been unconsciously internalized by the research community. Or, perhaps less insidiously, this absence of coverage in the literature may reflect the logistic difficulties sometimes involved in recruiting such minority group members for research.

In summary, the field of elderly sexuality itself is heterogeneous and diverse. Clinicians can expect only that their patients may come from a variety of backgrounds, with a myriad of sexual histories, current involvement in any number of sexual activities, and a potential range of physical health problems as well as a wide range of knowledge about these problems and their treatment. The benefit of knowledge of these diverse research findings is that we, as practitioners, will be better equipped to assist our elderly patients in coping with the physiological, demographic, and interpersonal changes they face with age.

# 2

# Knowledge of Elderly Sexuality

*One of the best predictors of an older adult's current level of sexual function-
ing is his or her past level of sexual functioning.*

When conducting an intake interview with an older adult, collecting information about that person's sexual history and current level of sexual activity is
often one of the last things on a health care provider's mind. Practitioners
usually have a brief, circumscribed period of time for this initial interview in
which they are consumed with assessing their older adult patient's mental
status, gathering pertinent medical information, building rapport, developing a
treatment plan, evaluating the underlying family or group dynamic, mobilizing
their patient's support system, and discussing the precipitating incident that
brought the patient for help. Because older adults often have a wealth of life
experience compared with many of their younger counterparts, gathering an
elderly patient's social history can be very time consuming. Difficulties in
gathering such information can be compounded further, particularly if the older
adult displays a sensory deficit or presents with an impaired mental status.
Despite the strenuous demands placed on a clinician when conducting a geriatric interview, it remains vital that the discussion of an elderly patient's sexual
activity, both current and historical, be granted high priority. One way that a
clinician can become better prepared to elicit such information is to become
familiar with some basic knowledge of elderly sexuality.

## SEXUAL BEHAVIOR ACROSS THE LIFE SPAN

Sexual behavior and its related goals, frequencies, types, and expectations
all can be expected to change throughout the life span. Among adolescents,
sexual behavior can provide a formal sense of identity, an opportunity to test
limits, an experience of emotional intimacy, and the chance to explore and
become comfortable with one's own body. For young adults in their 20s and 30s,
sexual behavior can provide an outlet for tension, opportunities for recreation

and pleasure, the expression of love and intimacy, the consummation of a marriage, and last, but certainly not least, the ability to become parents. Psychobiology suggests that sexual behavior among young adults serves the primary purpose of procreation and the solidification of pair bonds. Sex was biologically designed to "feel good" in order to promote childbearing and child rearing among healthy adults. In midlife, with the advent of menopause for women and some parallel hormonal changes in men, the biological goals of sexual behavior appear to change. Sexuality generally does not lead to parenthood; the pleasure, emotional intimacy, individual expression, and the desire to satisfy individual, familial, and societal expectations typically take precedence as the primary motivating factors for sexual behavior.

In late life, as compared with early adulthood and midlife, sexual activity enters a new realm in which its expression is related more directly to the personal motivation, needs, and satisfaction of the participants. Sexual activity in late life may be associated with desires to:

- Foster emotional intimacy
- Experience and enjoy physical pleasure
- Satisfy continuing biological urges
- Assert independence and to experiment with new things
- Feel youthful
- Challenge societal myths and stereotypes
- Reestablish a sexual identity
- Heighten bodily awareness
- Engender comfort and familiarity with a changing body

Issues of privacy, physical health, and the availability of a partner may become an even greater factor in the expression of sexual behavior for older adults. Even though clinicians and researchers often focus on the actual rates of sexual intercourse among older adults, it remains even more important to remember that the motivating (and limiting) factors for sexual relations among older adults may be *similar to or very different from* those of their younger counterparts.

## FREQUENCY AND TYPES OF SEXUAL BEHAVIORS

What Is Average and What Is Normal?

In discussing the relative frequency with which older adults engage in sexual activity, it becomes vital to make the distinction between "average" frequencies and types of behavior and "normal" frequencies and types of behavior. As among other age groups and subject populations, it is vital that both patients and practitioners understand the difference between average and normal participation rates. Average frequencies simply represent our best guess at a numerical mean for a specific sexual behavior, based on a specific sample of older adults using a specific research methodology. For example, Starr and Weiner (1981) reported that the participants in their study aged 80 years and older engaged in sexual intercourse 1.2 times per week, on average. However, these figures tell us nothing about whether these particular older adults were satisfied with their sexual relationships, whether they desired more or less sexual contact, and whether or not they had consistent access to a consenting sexual partner. In other words, what is "normal" or personally acceptable to one older adult may or may not be personally acceptable to another.

Unfortunately, many patients regard clinical averages as a benchmark that they must match or exceed in order to demonstrate that they are aging well. What is normal about elderly sexuality must be assessed on a case-by-case basis, with substantial emphasis placed on the perceptions, feelings, and expectations of the older adult in question. Patients often express incredible relief when they learn from their health care provider that the number that they read in a magazine article indicating how often they "should be having sex each week" does not indicate what is normal for them. Productive collaborative work between patient and practitioner begins when patients are able to focus on the nature and quality of their own sexual relationships instead of the relations that they believe they should be having in order to meet some primarily arbitrary, normal standard.

## Alfredo

Alfredo was a 76-year-old, decorated Air Force veteran of World War II. He attended group therapy at a day hospital program for older adults in order to help him work through residual issues from posttraumatic stress disorder. During the war, Alfredo was one of the few men to survive an unexpected enemy attack on his squadron. He interpreted this event as a divine sign that he was specially chosen to survive. This narcissistic interpretation of events helped him to assuage his guilt and to proceed through life with confidence, but also at a costly emotional price. Alfredo was particularly fearful of aging because "such a special person as myself should be allowed to remain on this earth for as long as possible." Regardless of the weather, Alfredo always seemed to wear his leather bomber jacket. He spoke daily about his vigorous exercise routine, feeling "as healthy as a horse," and still being lucky enough to have all of his hair. Although many of Alfredo's peers from the group therapy hospital program were irritated by his need to flaunt his wealth, status, and health, they tolerated his displays as if they knew that he could not easily tolerate this perceived, narcissistic injury of aging.

Unlike his peers in group therapy, his 72-year-old wife, Aleni, was less tolerant of Alfredo's narcissistic displays. Aleni sometimes traveled to the hospital with her husband for treatment team meetings and occasional couples sessions. In contrast to her husband, Aleni appeared comfortable with her own aging. She appeared happy and confident with her healthy and slightly plump figure. However, she sometimes appeared overly tired, particularly on the days after Alfredo insisted that they take a strenuous sightseeing trip or bike ride. Aleni also admitted to the staff psychologist that her husband was equally demanding in their bedroom. Aleni admitted that although she was pleased that her husband found her attractive and sexy, she sometimes wondered whether he really wanted to make love to her, or if he just wanted to prove something to himself.

When asked to broach the subject as a couple, Alfredo remarked that he just wanted to engage in sex with his wife as much as everybody else. When asked how he knew what "everybody else" did, he spoke about an article that he read in a popular men's health magazine. The article presented the results from a reader's poll in which the few elderly men who responded reported that they had sexual intercourse three times a week on average. Alfredo was highly motivated to remain as healthy, sexy, and competitive as the other elderly men. Although it certainly was not possible to address Alfredo's core narcissistic issues in a few couples session, Alfredo was able to understand that this average number of three essentially was arbitrary. When asked directly, Alfredo also noted that the article did not provide any information about whether these men who engaged in sex many times a week were satisfied with their physical or emotional relationships. The social worker further explained that the elderly men who chose to answer a survey for this young men's health magazine probably felt pressured to artificially inflate the number of times that they had sex each week.

More importantly, Aleni was able to tell her husband that she only wanted to have sex with him when they *both* wanted to feel close. With support from the psychologist, she was able to assert her rights to her own body. She told Alfredo that she would think more of him as a man if they had sex less often, but with more emotion and intensity instead of "just going through the motions so you can say you had it with me." She told him that she wanted to be a special part of his life, and not just some number that he had to live up to. The psychologist was able to draw a parallel to Alfredo's combat experience; she remarked that while Alfredo was very proud of how many enemy kills he had painted on the side of his aircraft, his wife wanted to be more than just a number to him in his own private war against aging. Alfredo initially balked at the idea, but soon recognized that his wife was being honest and forthright. He learned that his wife based his masculinity and youthfulness on the quality, and not the quantity, of their sexual relations. He also reported that he might feel more relaxed knowing that there was one less area in his life in which he had to measure up to some youthful standard in order to prove that he was special.

Introductory Research Findings

Despite the necessity of evaluating older adults' sexual behavior on an individual basis, a number of research studies do provide valuable information about general trends in sexual relations across the life span, and about the factors that are most predictive of sexual activity in later life. Again, emphasis should be placed on the fact that these research studies only highlight general trends, and that they do not indicate absolute ideals or expectations for elderly adults. What the findings of these studies do offer, however, is a wealth of information that contradicts the commonly held stereotype that older adults are asexual beings who do not participate in or desire sexual relations.

The first empirical studies to provide information about the sexual practices of older adults were conducted in the 1950s by Kinsey and his colleagues (Kinsey, Pomeroy, & Martin, 1948; Kinsey, Pomeroy, Martin, & Gebhard, 1953). It is notable that before this time, the sexual life of older adults was virtually unexplored in any scientific way. Societal prohibitions against the discussion of such topics certainly influenced the overall lack of research prior to this time, and led to an uproar among some segments of the public when these landmark studies' results were released. What Kinsey and his colleagues revealed was that among their sample of community living older adults, men over the age of 60 engaged in intercourse slightly more than once a week on average, with no sudden decline in sexual activity related to aging. Women over the age of 60 were found to engage in intercourse less frequently than their male counterparts, but with similar patterns of sexual behavior to those reported in their late teenage years. In the mid-1960s, Masters and Johnson (1966) also pronounced that men and women were biologically capable of engaging in sexual intercourse at any age.

Another series of researchers presented more detailed information regarding older adults' sexual behaviors during the mid-1970s and 1980s. George and Weiler (1981) recruited more than 340 elderly husbands and wives in a longitudinal study of sexual behavior. Excluding the effect of losing a partner by widowhood, the frequency of sexual activity among these elderly men and women remained remarkably stable over the 6-year study period. These spouses reported that they engaged in sexual intercourse between one and two times a week on average. Pfeiffer and Davis (1972) found that elderly women were more likely to engage in sexual relations if they were married. Specifically, an elderly woman's marital status, particularly whether she was divorced or single, was a better predictor of a decrease in her reported frequency of sexual intercourse than was her age itself. Although this finding appears remarkably obvious, it marked a drastic and important change in the way in which sex researchers began to interpret their basic frequency reports of sexual intercourse among elderly adults. Researchers, like clinicians, began to focus on some of the individual aspects of older adults that made them more or less likely to engage in specific types of sexual behavior. In other words, understanding the context in which an older person's sexual expression takes place began to take precedence over the acquisition of absolute numbers or base rates.

Other investigators also began to explore elderly sexuality beyond the singular act of intercourse. Butler and Lewis (1976) indicated that the sexual behaviors engaged in by elderly persons often encompassed more than intercourse, and that older adults often placed greater emphasis on cuddling, fondling, and mutual manual stimulation. Botwinick (1984) also expressed the importance of examining sexual gratification in regard to a variety of sexual behaviors among older adults, including self-stimulation. However, empirical findings regarding the numbers of elderly adults who engage in masturbation have varied greatly. For example, Starr and Weiner (1981) revealed that approximately one-half of the elderly participants in their study engaged in masturbation on a regular basis. In contrast, the majority of elderly participants in a study conducted by Wasow and Loeb (1979) reported that they refrained from self-stimulation, primarily out of religious concerns and an overall lack of privacy in an institutional setting. In sum, the few studies that did examine the extent to which older adults engaged in masturbation varied widely in their selection of subjects and the extent to which they addressed contextual issues (e.g., availability of a partner, religious beliefs and prohibitions), and their subsequent findings appear just as varied.

Current Research Findings

Although prior studies of elderly sexuality appear to be somewhat simplistic in the presentation of their findings, these researchers' willingness to explore a previously taboo topic provided the necessary impetus for more current and extensive examinations of elderly adults' sexual behavior. Matthias et al. (1997) present some of the most current information available about sexual activity among older adults. Their study is unique in that these researchers went beyond a basic assessment of base rates, and explored important, related issues of physical health, mental health, and sexual satisfaction. The study's sample was comprised of more than 1200 community living adults over the age of 65.

Perhaps the most striking, overall finding that emerged from the Matthias investigation was that although 30% of their elderly adults reported that they engaged in sexual activity during the past month, more than double this number, or 65%. of the elderly people in the total sample reported that they were satisfied or very satisfied with their current level of sexual activity or overall lack of sexual activity. Although more of the sexually active participants were younger, healthy, educated, married men, it appears that current sexual involvement is not necessarily a requirement for satisfaction with one's level of sexual activity. Results from these studies also suggest that engaging in sexual activity is not a guarantee of personal satisfaction. In some cases, sexual satisfaction and participation in sexual activity may be completely unrelated. This is an important concept for both patients and practitioners alike. Pervasive messages from our highly sexualized and youth-oriented society suggest that sexual satisfaction is reserved only for those who are currently and actively involved in a sexual relationship.

*Availability of a Partner.* Regarding the factors that are most predictive of whether an elderly person will be sexually active or not, Matthias et al. (1997) found that different aspects of the elderly participants' lives curtailed their participation in sexual activity. They discovered that elderly men and women responded differently to life stressors in terms of how they impacted on their sex lives. For example, marriage appears to be a significant predictor for sexual activity among elderly women, but not for elderly men. Among women, being single, widowed, or divorced meant that they were less likely to have an active sex life than their married counterparts.

A variety of factors might account for this difference in marital status as a predictor of sexual activity. First, our society maintains a double standard that men are hypersexual beings who require sexual outlets, and that while it is more acceptable to satisfy those sexual needs within the context of marriage, seeking sexual gratification outside of marriage is tolerated and sometimes viewed as exciting or accepted. The vast majority of prostitutes are women, who often work for married, male clients. Women, on the other hand, are expected to honor their marriage vows for their entire lives. A female adulterer typically is viewed with contempt, as an ungrateful and selfish spouse.

Additionally, the numbers of single elderly women greatly exceed the numbers of single elderly men. Women have a longer life span than men, and tend to marry men who are older than them. Because of basic laws of supply and demand, it is much easier for an elderly man to seek out a romantic or sexual relationship with a single elderly woman than it is for her to establish such a relationship with a single elderly man. Many older adult men in nursing homes, for example, find that they are not used to all of the attention that they receive from the multitude of single women in their midst. One elderly gentleman in a Florida retirement community took five elderly women at a time with him for breakfast at a local restaurant. Another five women had to wait their turn to go with him to lunch. One of these women was quoted wryly as saying, "Well, who am I to hurt his feelings and turn down a free lunch?" Another elderly woman regarded the situation plaintively and replied, "Sometimes you've got to take what you can get." Clinicians certainly must be aware of the self-esteem issues that come into play in such highly competitive environments.

*Physical Health.*   Another factor that is related to sexual activity among elderly adults is physical health. Older adults suffering from arthritis, high blood pressure, heart disease, stroke, diabetes, and kidney problems were found to engage in less sexual activity than those older adults who suffered from fewer of these chronic ailments (Matthias et al., 1997). Physical disability, in relation to functional status, also was related to engagement in sexual activity. Older adults who reported that they had difficulty getting in and out of bed, bathing themselves, and getting dressed and undressed had fewer sexual interludes than those who were independently mobile. Although this finding certainly is not surprising, it can provide relief to older adults who are suffering from medical problems; they learn that they are not alone or unique in their plight. In other words, it is normal for an elderly person who suffers from physical disabilities to engage in sexual behavior with lesser frequency than an elderly person in the best of health. However, it also is vital that older adults who suffer from physical illness and disabilities know that such difficulties do not automatically preclude them from satisfying, enjoyable, and frequent sexual relations if they so choose.

*Biological Age.*   Among couples who are married, age does appear to be related to overall frequency of sexual intercourse (Call et al., 1995). A recent study of more than 13,000 married couples nationwide revealed that sexual intercourse took place at least once in the past month among:

96% of those aged 19–24
92% of those aged 30–34

83% of those aged 50–54
57% of those aged 65–69
27% of those aged 75+

The couples also differed significantly by age group in terms of the average number of times they made love per month. The 19- to 24-year-olds had intercourse an average of 11.7 times per month; the 30- to 34-year-olds, 8.5 times per month; the 50- to 54-year-olds, 5.5 times per month; the young-old adults aged 65–69, 2.4 times per month; and the oldest-old adults aged 75 and older, 0.8 time per month. A detailed analysis of the 75+ age group revealed that although the average rate of sexual intercourse was less than once a month for all of the couples in this age group, the 27% of those oldest-old couples who were sexually active had sex an average of three times each month.

Like Matthias et al. (1997), Call et al. (1995) imagined that physical health was a better predictor of sexual activity than the formal nature of the relationship itself. However, multiple regression equations demonstrated that the decline in sexual activity and frequency among the older adults in their nationwide sample was not solely the result of an increase in physical illness and poor health; age alone appeared to play a significant role. Even among elderly married couples who have two healthy, consenting partners, the average frequency of sexual intercourse declines steadily with age. But, one can expect that even among the oldest-old, a relatively high level of sexual activity (or virtual inactivity) can be a normal part of an elderly person's life. Greater variability in sexual expression, not an inevitable cessation in sexual activity, appears to be the norm with aging. It also remains unchallenged that despite societal myths, older adults often remain satisfied with their sexuality, whether they are currently sexually active or not, and that elderly adults often possess sexual urges and interests late into the final decades of life.

What Is Abnormal?

Although anecdotal reports exist to substantiate that older adults engage in fetishes, bondage, bisexuality, cross-dressing, ménage à trois, and other deviations from culturally traditional sexual norms, virtually no research findings exist regarding the frequencies or predictors of these behaviors. What becomes more important when dealing with an elderly patient who presents with some deviant sexual behavior is to determine to what extent this behavior is abnormal, and whether attempts should be made to help the patient change this behavior. As in work with younger clients, it is important that clinicians not project their own values and expectations into their evaluation of a specific sexual activity or relationship. Important aspects to consider include:

- Is this behavior hurtful or harmful to the elderly person?
- Is this behavior hurtful or harmful to other people?
- Does this behavior disrupt the patient's daily functioning?
- Does this behavior disrupt the older person's interpersonal relationships?
- Is this behavior illegal?
- Are there violations of privacy or consent for other people?

- Does this behavior run counter to the patient's religious beliefs?
- Is involvement in this behavior ego syntonic or ego dystonic?
- Does performing this behavior put the patient at high risk for acquiring sexually transmitted illnesses such as AIDS?

Discussing involvement in such intensely private behaviors requires tact and sensitivity, regardless of the age of the patient. Many older adults are from a cohort in which sexual deviance, much less traditional sexual behavior, is considered an embarrassing topic to discuss even with health care professionals. Clinicians can expect that if an elderly patient does broach the subject of potentially deviant sexual behavior (e.g., voyeurism, bondage), it probably indicates a high level of trust in the professional relationship and the high level of stress and discomfort that the patient probably wants to alleviate.

### Anna

Anna, a 68-year-old married woman, was in weekly psychotherapy for treatment of moderately severe clinical depression. About 6 months into treatment, Anna had begun to gain the weight that she had lost, to develop some same-sex friendships outside of her marriage, to exercise on a weekly basis, and to become more assertive with her adult children about not wanting to baby-sit her grandson on a full time basis. The transference in the therapeutic relationship was positive and Anna had begun to engage in more, appropriate self-disclosure with each subsequent session. Once Anna's mood began to stabilize, she and her therapist began to explore other issues.

In her next session, with only a few minutes remaining in the therapy hour, Anna announced quietly that she had a secret that she wanted to share. She said that she had never told anyone else about it, either inside or outside of her family, and that she was very hesitant to talk about it. Her therapist suggested, "Well, because you feel so hesitant about telling this secret, maybe it would be easier to start by telling me about how you think you would feel if you told me about it, or what you think my reaction would be." Anna sighed and responded, "Well ... I guess I am afraid that you would think I am a terrible wife ... and that there is something really wrong with my husband." Her therapist retorted, "Even if I were to think that way, which I'm not sure I would, would that really be so terrible?" Anna smiled sheepishly and then frowned. She looked down at the floor, and said that a few months ago she walked into the master bedroom without knocking, and found her husband standing in front of the bureau, looking in the mirror, wearing a pair of her panties and one of her bras.

Anna kept looking at the ground, and said that she knew then that her husband must "be a queer ... a homo." She balled her hand into a fist and pounded it against her leg. Her gaze remained fixed on the ground. Anna began to cry and said, "It makes me feel so sick.... After it happened, Curt got dressed and ran out after me. He tried to tell me that he never wanted me to see him that way, that he was still a man, that he still loved me. I haven't really talked about it with him. We just pretend like things are going along as usual ... I mean, we haven't made love much in the past few years anyway; I guess this is part of the reason why.

I'm surprised he could force himself on me all of those years ... I mean, if he really didn't like women after all ... maybe he just wanted to 'do the right thing' and have children. I thought ...." Anna's voice grew thick and she began to sob.

Anna's therapist asked her if she would like to know what her husband's behavior was called. After nodding yes, Anna was told that her husband was engaging in *cross-dressing.* Anna looked up and said, "So there is a name for this ... thing he does, or they do?" Her therapist decided that additional information regarding her husband's behavior was warranted before delving into the emotional baggage associated with it, in order to dispel any additional myths. Anna's therapist continued, "Cross-dressing is when a man wears women's clothing in order to help feel aroused. Sometimes these men wear only women's underwear, and sometimes under their own clothes. The other important thing to know about this behavior is that most of the men who engage in cross-dressing are not homosexual or 'queer,' but heterosexual; they love women and find women sexually attractive, not men." Anna sat up a little straighter in her chair and asked, "So, you mean that Curt isn't gay or queer or whatever?" Her therapist responded, "It is more likely that he is not.... Now, you just told me something very important that you had kept a secret for a very long time, and we have only a few minutes left in our session and we will have to stop very soon. I think it's important that we wrap up and prepare to talk more about it next time.... Is this the reaction you thought you would have—that you thought I would have?"

It is notable that Anna missed her next two appointments. When asked matter of factly about her absence, Anna was able to articulate, "I guess I wasn't ready to talk about it just yet." Her therapy changed dramatically as the original precipitant to her depression was revealed, and Anna began to express her anger, fear, humiliation, and concerns about her husband's behavior. She also began to discuss adjunctive couples therapy in order to discuss Curt's behavior and its effect on her. (Anna said, "Why does he want to do that? I mean, that's sickening to me ... aren't I good enough for him to want me the way I am?" Anna's therapist also was able to provide important factual information about fetishes and the ways in which they are formed (e.g., the initiation of Curt's cross-dressing probably had little or nothing to do with Anna, and it may have begun even before he knew her).

In this case, Anna was able to discuss her feelings openly and to become angry about Curt's behavior instead of remaining paralyzed by it. It also was crucial that Anna's therapist did not become "paralyzed" in session over this revelation with her own countertransference; Anna's therapist herself was shocked that her first encounter with cross-dressing occurred in the context of therapy with an elderly couple. Whether a patient is younger or older, therapists and patients alike benefit from a thorough knowledge base of sexual behavior.

## A SELF-TEST FOR KNOWLEDGE

Based on the groundbreaking work of Charles White (1982), the Aging Sexual Knowledge and Attitudes Scale (ASKAS) has been used extensively among adult children of older adults, college students, health care providers, nursing home staff members, health care educators, and elderly persons themselves. Although it has been used primarily in research settings, it also can be employed successfully as a valuable educational tool for older adult patients. Asking an elderly couple to complete the knowledge section of the scale separately, and to then score their answers jointly often allows for a discussion of previously taboo topics. It also allows the practitioner to gain insight into the knowledge base of her clients. Many patients admit relief when they learn that some of the very stereotypes that they had ascribed to were false. Others realize for the first time that it is acceptable to discuss intimate sexual issues and concerns with their health care provider. This 35-item knowledge subtest of the ASKAS can be administered as a self-report paper-and-pencil test, or as a clinician-administered interview. This assessment instrument employs nonscientific language, and is suitable for elderly patients who have acquired less than a high school education. Presented in the appendix at the end of this chapter, the knowledge section of the ASKAS can be used as a self-test for clinicians as well. Some selected items from this knowledge section will be reviewed here.

## The Knowledge Section of the ASKAS

2. Males over the age of 65 typically take longer to attain an erection of their penis than do younger males. TRUE. Because of changes in the internal structure of the penis over the age of 60 (i.e., most men develop more venous blood vessels that are larger in diameter), most elderly men require increased blood flow to the penis in order to attain an erection. It takes more time for an older man to have an erection, related in large part to the increased time it takes to provide increased blood flow to the penis. Many older men also find that they need more tactile stimulation in order to attain a full erection.

4. The firmness of erection in aged males is often less than that of younger persons. TRUE. Because of changes in the blood flow to the penis, older adult males often have a less firm and erect erection than younger males, sometimes impeding their ability to penetrate a female partner during intercourse. Some estimates suggest that up to one-half of men over the age of 75 have some degree of erectile dysfunction (Kaiser, 1991).

7. The older female may experience painful vaginal intercourse due to reduced elasticity of the vagina and reduced vaginal lubrication. TRUE. Many older adult women benefit from the use of water-based lubricants such as KY jelly in order to alleviate any discomfort during intercourse associated with vaginal dryness. Some researchers suggest that up to two-thirds of elderly women experience discomfort during intercourse, related primarily to a lack of lubrication. The more positive aspect of this finding is that the problem is usually readily treatable with over-the-counter lubricants, and prescription lubricants and hormone therapies.

8. Sexuality is typically a lifelong need. TRUE. Masters and Johnson (1966) were among the first researchers to point out that older adults have as much interest in and need for sexual contact as their younger counterparts. Even

though an older person can no longer produce offspring, the underlying biological urge to engage in sexual (and sensual) activity does not appear to diminish significantly with age. In the classic study by Bretschneider and McCoy (1988), healthy elderly men and women were found to engage in sexual activity well into their 90s and even past their 100th birthday.

9. Sexual behavior in older people increases the risk of heart attack. FALSE. Unless an older adult is under a physician's orders to limit his or her physical activity, sexual activity can be actively pursed by older adults without fear of life-threatening exertion. Among healthy older adults, sexual activity can provide some of the benefits of cardiovascular exercise. There also is evidence that sexual activity in older persons has beneficial physical effects on the participants. Increased blood flow to the genital area can provide an older women with increased vaginal lubrication and can provide an older man with more sustained erections in future sexual relations.

11. The relatively more sexually active younger people tend to become the relatively more sexually active older people. TRUE. One of the best predictors of an elderly person's sexual activity is his or her prior level of sexual activity. Men and women who did not engage in sexual relations in their younger years are less likely to engage in sexual relations during their later years (Call et al., 1995). Of course, availability of a partner and physical health, among other factors, can limit this trend.

13. Sexual activity may be psychologically beneficial to older person participants. TRUE. Many older adults cite that they enjoy their sexual relationships even more than they did when they were younger. Others point out that even though they may engage in sexual activities less frequently than they did when they were younger, they cherish and enjoy them more. It also is common to hear older adults mention that they typically feel more comfortable with their partner, and no longer have "unrealistic expectations" about the sex act.

16. Prescription drugs may alter a person's sex drive. TRUE. A variety of prescription medications for depression, blood pressure, and diabetes can negatively impact on an older person's level of sexual interest and level of sexual functioning. Clinicians should be aware of all medications that an elderly person is taking.

21. The most common determinant of the frequency of sexual activity in older couples is the interest or lack of interest of the husband in a sexual relationship with his wife. TRUE. For married older adults, studies do suggest that the rates of sexual intercourse are determined primarily by the interest level of the husband. It remains unclear, however, to what extent this can be accounted for by a cohort effect. In this current elderly cohort, the husband is primarily responsible for making sexual advances; "good wives" were unlikely to initiate sexual behavior. In this cohort, the elderly wife also has been inculcated with the expectation that "a good wife does not say 'no' to her husband." Both of these beliefs further increase the likelihood that the frequency of sexual activity among current elderly couples is influenced primarily by the husband's level of interest and desire.

22. Barbiturates, tranquilizers, and alcohol may lower the sexual arousal levels of aged persons and interfere with sexual responsiveness. TRUE. Many over-the-counter medications and substances can impact on an older adult's sexual functioning. Because older adults metabolize alcohol more slowly than younger adults, even one or two alcoholic drinks can negatively impact on sexual function. Heavy consumption of cigarettes also may diminish sexual desire, and nicotine also has been related to impotence among elderly men.

23. Sexual disinterest in aged persons may be a reflection of a psychological state of depression. TRUE. One of the most common symptoms of depression is a loss of interest in sexual activity. Among older adults without available sexual partners, it is still appropriate (and recommended) that clinicians ask that older adult if her or his own interest in sexuality has changed. One might ask, "Even if you haven't been engaged in sexual relations for a few years, do you find yourself thinking about sex less frequently than you used to in the past few months?"

28. Fear of the inability to perform sexually may bring about an inability to perform sexually in older males. TRUE. Impotence has been known to be initiated by psychological causes. Fear of intimacy and fear of attaining an erection have been identified as some of these common concerns. "Widower's syndrome" also been identified. In this syndrome, a recent widower who is not yet emotionally prepared for intimacy with another woman (particularly if he had been married in a relationship spanning many decades), experiences impotence with a newly introduced female partner. However, clinicians must first rule out organic causes for impotency among their older adult male patients.

29. The ending of sexual activity in old age is most likely and primarily due to social and psychological causes rather than biological and physical causes. TRUE. Many of the physical problems associated with aging can be addressed. Even older adults with chronic illness can engage in a variety of sexual behaviors if they so choose. Many older adults cease to become sexual beings simply from perceived societal pressures and stereotypes. Societal myths suggest that older adults are asexual beings who are not entitled to the benefits and joys of sexuality (and sensuality) that seem to belong exclusively to the young.

35. Masturbation in older males and females has beneficial effects on the maintenance of sexual responsiveness. TRUE. For men, masturbation can improve blood flow to the penis and help prevent future incidents of impotence. For women, masturbation has been shown to increase blood flow to the vaginal area and promote premenopausal levels of lubrication. Some clinicians have successfully "prescribed" masturbation to elderly women, who later reported that they were able to experiment with and enjoy self-stimulation for the first time in their lives after receiving approval from their health care provider.

Reviewing aspects of elderly sexuality is vital. Studies show that health care providers and health care educators (Glass & Webb, 1995), as well as elderly persons themselves (Adams, Rojas-Comero, & Clayton, 1990; Smith & Schmall, 1983), often have limited knowledge of elderly sexuality. As clinicians, we owe it to our patients and ourselves to be informed about elderly sexuality.

## INTAKE ASSESSMENT

Although many elderly patients, like their younger counterparts, seem to reveal important aspects of their sex life only after they have been in treatment for an extended period of time, most information about an older person's sex life can be gathered effectively during the initial intake interview. It is important that clinicians place value on this information, and recognize that obtaining such information represents much more than just finding about how many times a week their patient has sex with the significant other. Asking our elderly patients about their sex lives provides us with valuable opportunities early in treatment to discuss and assess:

- Emotional intimacy
- Body image
- Physical health
- Medical history
- Self-esteem
- Quality of interpersonal relationships
- Ascribed sex roles
- Sexual identity and orientation
- Attitudes toward aging
- Knowledge of elderly sexuality
- Religion
- Sense of humor

How to Gather Information

Interviewing an older adult about sexual matters can pose unique problems as well opportunities. Many older adults are reticent to discuss such personal matters without proper groundwork by the clinician. Before addressing issues of sexuality and sexual behavior, it often can be helpful to simply ask the patient permission to inquire about such matters (e.g., "May I ask you some questions about your love and sex life?") Asking the patient for such permission can instill a sense of respect and concern; the patient is given control in a potentially anxiety-provoking situation. Another tactic is to present the questions as part of the standard interview that is used with all patients who come to the clinic. Likening sexual information to medical information also can allow elderly patients to feel more comfortable discussing such personal issues. In some cases, admitting that "it is not always an easy thing for physicians or patients to talk about, but it is important that we gather some information about your love and sex life" normalizes the stress and anxiety that an older person may feel about discussing sexual issues with a clinician.

When asking questions about sexual behaviors, it is important to word questions in "the affirmative." In other words, it is helpful to provide older adults with an opportunity to answer the question without appearing as though they are admitting something wrong, immoral, or embarrassing. For example, instead of asking, "How many affairs have you had?" it would be preferable to say, "Some people become unhappy in their marriages, for any number of reasons, and engage in extramarital affairs or seek out other lovers. Can you tell me about any affairs you may have had?" It also is beneficial to allow for humor in the process. Sometimes humor (on the part of the clinician or the patient) is appropriate and helps to dispel tension.

Requisite Information

It is important to gather a variety of information regarding an older adult's sexuality. Sometimes it helps to have a checklist or other rough guideline available during the course of the clinical interview. Some relevant questions for both older men and women include (see also Galindo & Kaiser, 1995):

- What would you consider a satisfactory sex life? Some people are satisfied while other people are dissatisfied with their sex lives. How do you feel about your sex life?
- How long has it been since you have engaged in any sexual activity?
- Do you have any current sexual partners? Do you have an exclusive relationship or do either of you have other partners as well? (Gather activity about the sex, numbers, and potential high-risk behavior of the partners such as prostitution or drug use.)
- Does your religion influence how you feel about sex, or influence your current sexual activities in any way? Can you tell me about your religious views?
- Having sex means different things to different people. For some people it means having sexual intercourse and to others it means holding hands. What different types of intimate sexual activity [vaginal intercourse, oral sex, anal intercourse, petting, cuddling, holding hands] do you engage in?
- How often do you masturbate or touch yourself to feel good? How do you feel about it? (This is often a good opportunity to tell an older adult about the potential emotional and physical benefits of masturbation.)
- As people age, they sometimes experience pain or discomfort during sexual intercourse. Do you ever experience such pain or discomfort?
- The average person experiences some kind of sexual difficulties at some point in life. Could you tell me about any trouble or problems that you, or a partner of yours, may have had in the past? Do you have any concerns about your sexual behavior or functioning right now that you could tell me about?
- Some people experience changes in their body as they age, either slowly over time or more suddenly through illness or surgery. How do you feel about your body? How does your partner feel about your body?
- Do you use any lubricating gels or liquids when you engage in sex? What kind do you use? (Does the elderly adult use something inappropriate like an oil based lubricant such as Vaseline, or does she use something water soluble like KY jelly?)

- Do you have any concerns or worries about your sexual performance?
- (Even if you have not had sexual relations lately) have you been thinking more or less about sex than you typically have in the last few months?
- Do you feel you have enough privacy for the sexual activities that you want to engage in?
- Is there anything about your sex life that you wish were different?
- How easy or difficult is it for you to talk about your sexual behavior with your partner? Your physician? With me right now? (You can inform patients that they are doing a wonderful job talking about such a personal topic, if in fact they are. This also can provide an opportunity to talk about how many people feel uneasy talking about sexual matters, and to empathize with their fears and concerns.)
- People often have questions they would like to ask about sex. Do you have some questions about sexual activity that you would like to ask me?

Some specific questions also should be directed to members of the opposite sex. For example, older women can be asked about potential discomfort during intercourse, and age of menopause. Men can be asked about their erections and their frequency of urination. Depending on the numbers of types of partners that both elderly men and women have (especially if high-risk behaviors are involved), pointed questions should be asked about condom use. Older people also should be asked if they know how to properly put on a condom, and whether they know that a new condom should be used for each subsequent act of intercourse. Many older adults underestimate their risk of contracting a sexually transmitted disease outside of a long-term monogamous relationship, and focus mainly on their freedom from fear of unwanted conception.

Because so many prescription and over-the-counter medications can be associated with a decrease in sexual desire and function (see Galindo & Kaiser, 1995), clinicians should make a concerted effort to gather detailed information about a patient's medication history. As gathering such medication information is already a prerequisite for a thorough geriatric intake, no additional time will be lost during an interview with an elderly patient who may (or may not) initially discuss concerns about changes in their sexual functioning. Because older adults typically take a large number of prescription and over-the-counter medications and because they may present with a decline in mental status, it may be difficult to get a proper assessment of daily medication intake. One way to circumvent these problems is to ask patients to bring a "brown bag" that contains all of their current medications with them to the intake interview. Names of medications, as well as the names of the prescribing physicians, can be taken directly from pill bottles. Important information also can be gleaned as to whether an elderly person is taking the medication as instructed on the label, whether he or she is noncompliant based on the number of pills remaining in the bottle, or whether he or she misunderstood the directions for administration in the first place. Many elderly people are surprised to learn that a variety of drugs, including those listed in Table 1, can interfere with sexual functioning.

TABLE 1.  Drugs that Can Impair Sexual Function
among Elderly Adults[a]

| Prescribed/used for | Drug | Common or trade name |
|---|---|---|
| Anxiety | Benzodiazepines | |
| Cancer | Chemotherapy agents | |
| Colds/flu | Antihistamines | |
| Epilepsy | Carbamazepine | Tegretol |
| | Ethosuximide | Zarontin |
| Glaucoma | Metoclopramide HCl | Reglan |
| High blood pressure | Clonidine HCl | Catapres |
| | Methyldopa | Aldomet |
| | Prazosin HCl | Minipress |
| | Spironolactone | Aldactone |
| Mood disorders | Antidepressants | Prozac, Zoloft, Paxil |
| Parkinson's disease | Carbidopa/levodopa | Sinemet |
| Recreation | Ethyl alcohol | Beer, wine, liquor |
| | Nicotine | Cigarettes, chew, snuff |
| | Narcotics | Cocaine, heroin |
| Schizophrenia | Antipsychotics | Haldol |
| Sedation (sleeping pills) | | |

[a]This table is in no way designed to be all-inclusive; any number of additional medications can impair sexual functioning.

## SUMMARY

Gathering information about an elderly patient's sex life is challenging, rewarding, and a requisite part of a geriatric intake interview. In order to make this practice more effective and efficient, clinicians themselves can become more informed about basic aspects of elderly sexuality. Some primary aspects of elderly sexuality are that older adults have been shown to be sexually active into the last decade of life. The best predictors of elderly people's sexual activity are their prior level of sexual activity and satisfaction, the availability of a partner, and their physical health. Many older adults themselves are uninformed about the physiological changes associated with aging and sexuality; many older adults do not know that impotence may be treatable or that masturbation can promote improved sexual lubrication in women. Many older adults, as well as health care providers, are not aware that commonly prescribed medications and over-the-counter drugs can significantly impair sexual function. Gathering information about an elderly patient's past and current sex life can reveal important information about close relationships, body image, knowledge of elderly sexuality, medical history, and self-esteem. As informed clinicians, the chance to discuss issues of sexuality with our elderly patients presents us with unique opportunities and benefits.

## APPENDIX

Knowledge Section of the ASKAS[a]

Answer Key: T = True; F = False; DK = Don't know

1.  **T**/F/DK    Sexual activity in aged persons is often dangerous to their health.
2.  **T**/F/DK    Males over the age of 65 typically take longer to attain an erection of their penis than do younger males.
3.  **T**/F/DK    Males over the age of 65 usually experience a reduction in intensity of orgasm relative to younger males.
4.  **T**/F/DK    The firmness of erection in aged males is often less than that of younger persons.
5.  **T**/F/DK    The older female (65+ years of age) has reduced vaginal lubrication secretion relative to younger females.
6.  **T**/F/DK    The aged female takes longer to achieve adequate vaginal lubrication relative to younger females.
7.  **T**/F/DK    The older female may experience painful vaginal intercourse due to reduced elasticity of the vagina and reduced vaginal lubrication.
8.  **T**/F/DK    Sexuality is typically a lifelong need.
9.  T/**F**/DK    Sexual behavior in older people increases the risk of heart attack.
10. T/**F**/DK    Most males over the age of 65 are unable to engage in sexual intercourse.
11. **T**/F/DK    The relatively more sexually active younger poeple tend to become the relatively more sexually active older people.
12. **T**/F/DK    There is evidence that sexual activity in older persons has beneficial physical effects on the participants.
13. **T**/F/DK    Sexual activity may be psychologically beneficial to older person participants.
14. T/**F**/DK    Most older females are sexually unresponsive.
15. T/**F**/DK    The sex urge typically increases with age in males over 65.
16. **T**/F/DK    Prescription drugs may alter a person's sex drive.
17. T/**F**/DK    Females, after menopause, have a physiologically induced need for sexual activity.
18. **T**/F/DK    Basically, changes with advanced age (65+) in sexuality involve a slowing of response time rather than a reduction of interest in sex.
19. **T**/F/DK    Older males typically experience a reduced need to ejaculate and hence may maintain an erection of the penis for a longer time than younger males.
20. T/**F**/DK    Older males and females cannot act as sex partners as both need younger partners for stimulation.
21. **T**/F/DK    The most common determinant of the frequency of sexual activity in older couples is the interest or lack of interest of the husband in a sexual relationship with his wife.

22. **T/F/DK** Barbiturates, tranquilizers, and alcohol may lower the sexual arousal levels of aged persons and interfere with sexual responsiveness.

23. **T/F/DK** Sexual disinterest in aged persons may be a reflection of a psychological state of depression.

24. **T/F/DK** There is a decrease in frequency of sexual activity with older age in males.

25. **T/F/DK** There is a greater decrease in male sexuality with age than there is in female sexuality.

26. **T/F/DK** Heavy consumption of cigarettes may diminish sexual desire.

27. **T/F/DK** An important factor in the maintenance of sexual responsivenss in the aging male is the consistency of sexual activity throughout his life.

28. **T/F/DK** Fear of the inability to perform sexually may bring about an inability to perform sexually in older males.

29. **T/F/DK** The ending of sexual activity in old age is most likely and primarily due to social and psychological causes rather than biological and physical causes.

30. **T/F/DK** Excessive masturbation may bring about an early onset of mental confusion and dementia in the aged.

31. **T/F/DK** There is an inevitable loss of sexual satisfaction in post-menopausal women.

32. **T/F/DK** Secondary impotence (or non-physiologically caused) increases in males over the age of 60 relative to younger males.

33. **T/F/DK** Impotence in aged males may literally be effectively treated and cured in many instances.

34. **T/F/DK** In the absence of severe physical disability, males and females may maintain sexual interest and activity well into their 80s and 90s.

35. **T/F/DK** Masturbation in older males and females has beneficial effects on the maintenance of sexual responsiveness.

*These items from the ASKAS appear from White (1982) with permission.

# 3

# Attitudes toward Elderly Sexuality

*Our youth-oriented culture views the process of aging as a tragic, narcissistic injury instead of as an opportunity for personal growth and change. Unfortunately, many older adults internalize and generalize these negative attitudes toward their own sexuality, and diminish or cease sexual expression out of fear, disgust, and shame. The attitudes that clinicians hold toward elderly sexuality also can influence their patients' attitudes toward elderly sexuality.*

After one considers the availability of a partner and general health status, one of the most important determinants of older adults' sexual activity is the positivity of their attitudes toward elderly sexuality. Attitudes toward elderly sexuality range from permissive to restrictive, curious to avoidant, and can be global or specific in relation to particular behaviors such as masturbation or sexuality within an institution. Different populations maintain different attitudes that differentially affect older adults. Health care providers including psychologists, psychiatrists, social workers, nurses, pharmacists, occupational therapists, and nutritionists all play a role in influencing an older adult's attitude toward elderly sexuality, either directly or indirectly. As clinicians, it is not sufficient to be aware of the attitudes toward elderly sexuality maintained by society and by our elderly patients themselves; we must also be cognizant of our own attitudes toward elderly sexuality. To some extent, it does not matter as much whether our own attitudes are permissive or restrictive. Our positive and negative reactions to our elderly patients can often serve as important diagnostic barometers for what is happening within the therapeutic alliance. The clinical issue at stake is whether we can observe our own attitudes and reactions to our elderly patients' sexuality, but maintain objective and neutral attitudes in our work with them.

## HOW ATTITUDES AFFECT BEHAVIOR

Within the social psychological literature, it has been documented consistently via rigorous research studies that attitudes are often linked to behavior. Although a number of factors can certainly moderate the relationship between an individual's attitude or feelings about something and his or her resulting behavior, clinicians often find that a patient's attitude about aging often influences his or her behavior in a variety of realms. Some elderly patients believe that aging is suggestive of forced retirement, a decline in physical health, an increase in sadness and depression, and a loss of value in our society. For many elderly patients, such negative attitudes toward aging are translated into a decline in sexual expression and a loss in an innate sense of sexuality.

## Geriatric Sexuality Breakdown Syndrome

Kaas (1981) was the first researcher to identify and categorize the potentially negative impact of aging on an older adult's sexuality. She called this process, in which the social environment of elderly adults becomes an overwhelming force for behavioral change and even for mental illness, Geriatric Sexuality Breakdown Syndrome. Kaas described it as an outcropping of Social Breakdown Syndrome (Kuypers & Bengston, 1973), that is, elderly people in a vicious cycle in which ageist societal attitudes become internalized. As a result, the elderly person begins to feel and act useless and helpless. Such apathy leads to further societal perceptions that elderly adults are mere hindrances, who require care and valuable societal resources without contributing anything in return. Unlike many Eastern societies, our individualized, Westernized society values independence, autonomy, and the related goods or services that an individual member of society can generate. Elderly adults, who typically retire from the workplace, are viewed as liabilities by many younger segments of society, rather than as a store of wisdom, experience, and reverence.

Kaas (1981) outlined a series of steps that take place when an elderly person undergoes this emotional and subsequent sexual breakdown. This series of events is presented in Table 2. Not all elderly adults appear to be impacted by

TABLE 2.   Geriatric Sexuality Breakdown Syndrome

| Step | Label | Manifestations |
|------|-------|----------------|
| 1 | Precondition susceptibility | Identity problems; diminished ego strength; changes in physiological sexual response |
| 2 | Dependence on available cues | Cues from sexual taboos and myths of geriatric sexlessness; few elderly role models |
| 3 | Societal labeling | "Dirty old man" and "indecent old woman" perceived as their own label if they engage in sexual behavior |
| 4 | Sick role | Role of perverse older person; perception of "sick," abnormal sexual desires |
| 5. | Learning of behaviors | Verbal disavowal of any sexual desire or activity; decrease in sexual activity |
| 6. | Atrophy of social skills | Loss of sexual performance skills for sexual excitement and enjoyment |
| 7. | Self-labeling/internalization | Self perception as "dirty old" man or woman; identification and acceptance of asexual status |

Geriatric Sexuality Breakdown Syndrome. The first condition that must be satisfied in order to initiate this syndrome is some kind of susceptibility to negative, societal influences. These factors may include identity problems or diminished ego strength, either through difficult transitions into retirement or a difficult adjustment to a chronic illness. Sometimes a change in sexual physiology (e.g., a reduction in response time or impotence related to a medical condition) can preclude the emergence of Geriatric Sexuality Breakdown Syndrome. In the second step of the syndrome, elderly adults rely on cues from their environment to rationalize their feelings and behavior. They receive messages from society at large in which older adults are sexless beings who are not capable of engaging in satisfying sexual relations. Other messages in the media about elderly sexuality are absent, simply because so few older adults, much less sexually active older adults, are available as role models.

In the third and fourth stages, elderly adults begin to accept these societal labels, and regard themselves as a "dirty old man" or "indecent old woman" if they seek out sexual contact or engage in sexual behavior. Society also introduces the role of a "sick elder," where sexual conduct among elderly adults is not just seen as unusual, it is viewed as perverse and pathological. In the fifth stage of the syndrome, an older adult feels pressured from society and his or her own internalized fears and limitations, and suddenly begins to report having "no interest" in sexuality. Such adults literally talk themselves out of their needs and desires for intimacy and sexual expression. A decrease in the frequency and types of sexual behavior follows.

In the sixth stage of this breakdown, the underlying skills for sexual enjoyment and arousal become diminished and sometimes lost. The interpersonal skills required to maintain sexual relations may wither and become obsolete, and the elder may manifest symptoms of apathy, depression, and even hostility and guilt. In the final stage of the syndrome, the elderly adult has internalized all of the negative attitudes espoused by society, and has reinforced these beliefs with his or her own decline in sexual activity, desire, and pleasure. The elderly adult has accepted the asexual status, and in effect has confirmed society's negative belief system. Kaas (1981) also reports that as pervasive as this syndrome is, clinicians can play a role in breaking this vicious cycle. The most critical aspect of intervention is assisting an elderly person in resisting society's negative attitudes and cues.

## Jayne

Jayne was a 78-year-old woman who had been divorced for more than 25 years. She was cognitively intact, and her only chronic illness was arthritis. Jayne required a walker to move about, but otherwise was able to drive, shop, tend to her apartment, and prepare her own meals. She had a small cadre of single women and married couples with whom she played bingo and attended church weekly. Jayne had begun psychotherapy during the past 2 months because she had begun to feel depressed about her increasing lack of mobility; she feared that her worsening rheumatoid arthritis might force her to give up driving soon. Jayne was most upset about not driving because it would increase her dependence on others, and because she feared it would limit her ability to socialize with others. When asked about those in her social circle, she admitted that one man from her church expressed interest in taking her to movies, going to a local diner, and taking a cruise. Jayne responded that there was no way she could negotiate a cruise ship, although she would certainly not become involved with this gentleman anyway.

When asked what she did not like about this suitor, Jayne responded that there was "nothing wrong with him." She described him as funny, vibrant, and active. She remarked that since he also was divorced for many years, she would not feel as though she were in "any type of competition" with his ex-wife. Puzzled by Jayne's resistance for companionship, her therapist asked her what was keeping her from enjoying this man's company. Jayne responded that it had been "a long time" since she had been with a man, and that she was afraid he would make sexual advances. When asked what exactly she was afraid of, Jayne reported that she was not so concerned about her arthritis inhibiting her sexuality, but was instead preoccupied with "what people would think." "After all," she said, "I am over 70 years old.... What kind of example would I be setting for the children at church? Old women don't prance around holding hands or kissing somebody much less. I don't know what I'm thinking about!"

Jayne clearly maintained a need for companionship and sexual intimacy (e.g., she certainly had given thought to engaging in sexual activities with this gentleman), but felt compelled by unspoken societal taboos to abort the relationship before it even got started. Only after Jayne was able to explore, and compare and contrast her own needs and desires with the inaccurate and limiting views of society, did she have enough confidence to accept a date with this elderly gentleman. She also was open to receiving education about some of the changes that may alter the sexual response through aging. At last report, their relationship had blossomed slowly both emotionally and sexually, and Jayne was able to enjoy a renewed sense of love and vitality.

## Some Research Findings

Research studies also show that among older adults themselves, attitudes toward their own sexuality are quite variable. Some psychoeducational programs have succeeded in increasing the knowledge base of older adults regarding sexual function (White & Catania, 1982), but with the caveat that many of the participants claimed that it did not change how they felt about specific sexual behaviors or their decisions to engage in sexual activities (Adams et al., 1990). Some older adults have been emphatic about their desire to avoid discussing elderly sexuality in its entirety (Adams et al., 1990), whereas other older adults have expressed great interest in learning more about elderly sexuality (Smith & Schmall, 1983).

Some researchers have suggested that a number of factors can influence one's attitude toward elderly sexuality. Among older adults, one's religious convictions appear to color attitudes toward elderly sexuality (Adams et al., 1990; Hillman & Stricker, 1994, 1996), and often quite specifically to generate restrictive attitudes toward sexual relations outside of marriage and to mastur-bation. Practitioners also appear to be influenced by their religious beliefs (Hillman & Stricker, 1994) and profess more negative and restrictive attitudes toward elderly sexuality as a result. Individuals with strong Catholic beliefs have often cited that masturbation (i.e., sexual activity that precludes the possi-bility of producing children) and sexual relations outside of marriage are sinful. One certainly must be aware and respectful of an elderly patient's religious views. The current cohort of older adults typically espouses more religiosity than the current cohort of middle-aged baby boomers, and a proper assessment of religious beliefs is a requisite part of any clinical interview.

As these research findings of attitudes toward elderly sexuality suggest, clinical practice demands that we be highly attuned to the needs, wants, and beliefs of our clients as individuals. While empirical research findings are vital in that they provide us with clear quantitative findings, they often minimize the unique, qualitative contributions of individual participants. This is where we, as clinicians, must regard empirical research as the foundation for our individ-ual patient interactions. Trust in our clinical skills, tempered with empirical knowledge, provides a solid foundation for dealing most effectively with issues of sexuality among older adult patients.

## ATTITUDES IN THE PATIENT–PRACTITIONER RELATIONSHIP

Whether taking a psychodynamic or cognitive–behavioral approach to ther-apy, clinicians from nearly every theoretical orientation accept that the quality of the relationship between the patient and practitioner prepares the foundation for all therapeutic work that follows. Trust, open communication, and empathy are required elements for the unfolding and working through of transference in the relationship as well as the completion of essential homework assignments. The quality of the patient–practitioner relationship is especially important in relation to issues of elderly sexuality. In order to generate such a positive therapeutic relationship, a number of potential stumbling blocks must be recog-nized and addressed.

### Countertransference

Many practitioners have strong emotional reactions to working with elderly patients, much less to working with elderly patients who are dealing with issues of sexuality. As clinicians, our own emotional reactions and attitudes toward our elderly patients can be the source of enhanced insight and diagnostic assessment, as well as the cause of therapeutic impasse and resistance in treat-ment. Countertransference to elderly patients can take many forms. Some of the more common, but certainly not all inclusive, countertransference reactions to working with elderly adults include:

- Fear of aging
- Fear of dying
- Counterphobic reactions to aging (e.g., Aging is so wonderful!)

- Desires to heal or rescue
- Curiosity
- Impatience
- Disgust
- Awe
- Reverence
- Wishes to be reunited with benevolent grandparents
- Wishes to be parented
- Wishes to be a parent or caretaker
- Exhibitionistic tendencies to appear vigorous and youthful
- Fear of intimacy
- Fear of loss
- Desires to experience history or another halcyon era

It also is common for clinicians to experience one or any combination of these feelings at any time during treatment. It also is quite normal and expected to have ambivalent, or contradictory, feelings when working with elderly patients. Many practitioners feel guilty or ashamed of their feelings of fear, disgust, or reverence. As we often tell our patients, having a variety of feelings is normal, to be expected, and to some extent beyond our control. What is within our control is how we process and respond to those feelings. We need to consider whether we act appropriately or inappropriately with our patients when such potentially powerful feelings arise.

Lorraine

To make matters more complicated, countertransference to an elderly patient can manifest itself both consciously and unconsciously (as with any patient). A therapist in training was working closely with a 76-year-old widow named Lorraine. Lorraine inspired feelings of awe and reverence in her therapist; she was feisty, outgoing, and determined to enjoy her life in spite of her arthritis, recent loss of her husband, a dwindling income, and rapidly failing eyesight. She always seemed to have a joke, a funny story, or tales of adventures to new places with friends each week. Yet, she still was able to talk about the loss of her husband and her range of new feelings in response to becoming a widow. Approximately 6 months into therapy, Lorraine had to schedule her weekly appointments at different times during the week in order to accommodate numerous trips to the hospital and to her physician's office for diagnostic tests. The medical team feared that Lorraine's glaucoma was worsening as a result of her high blood pressure. Lorraine's therapist also began to notice some subtle changes in her mental status that brought up a discussion of initiating neuropsychological testing in order to rule out multi-infarct dementia related to her dangerously high blood pressure. Lorraine's therapist's primary response was that her brave, outgoing patient could handle virtually anything, and that surely everything would turn out just fine.

Approximately two weeks later, Lorraine called her therapist one weekday afternoon and asked, "What happened to you yesterday? I started to get worried." What had happened was that Lorraine's therapist had forgotten to write down their rescheduled appointment time for the previous day, and had failed to show up for their session. Lorraine laughed about the incident and said, "Well, that's all right. You know me, I always like to get out of the house." When she discussed it with her supervisor, Lorraine's therapist realized that she had some unconscious motivation for "forgetting" about their appointment. Lorraine's apparent chink in her lively armor forced her therapist to consider that Lorraine, despite her positive mental outlook, was an elderly woman with serious medical problems. Lorraine's therapist did not want to acknowledge that her patient's increasing physician visits (1) interfered with the structure and intimacy that they had worked toward for months to foster and maintain, and (2) provided a cruel reminder that Lorraine may not have many years of independent living left as she had once believed. Lorraine's therapist also was able to acknowledge her own feelings of loss of control, namely, losing control over the treatment schedule and, more importantly, losing Lorraine both literally and figuratively if she were to have a more serious stroke.

Lorraine's therapist also was able to admit to herself that Lorraine's sudden change in appearance, from a tanned, fit and trim older woman who wore tasteful clothing and colorful makeup to a pale, hunched figure who had little energy to shop for trendy clothes or to see well enough to apply her makeup properly, quite simply, frightened her. These changes made her think about her own aging. Lorraine's therapist often thought that when she grew old herself, she would choose to be youthful and active, just like Lorraine. Lorraine had been the healthiest patient in her caseload, compared to numerous other older adults who used walkers, had speech impediments, were housebound, or suffered from Alzheimer's disease. Lorraine's therapist had placed her own high expectations of Lorraine and her excellent physical and emotional health above her own patient's need for expression, change, and acceptance.

Supervision was helpful in allowing Lorraine's therapist to accept that her countertransferential feelings were a normal and expected part of the treatment process. She was able to realize that glamorizing Lorraine as a function of her own phobic reaction to aging was preventing a vital discussion of aging and physical decline with her patient when she needed it most. Lorraine's therapist also was able to stop feeling guilty about her own lapse in memory, and to use this incident as a catalyst in their next session to address issues of trust, loss, and change. In other words, acting out on the part of the therapist does not mean that the therapeutic alliance is ruptured permanently. Often, it can be interpreted and used as an important tool within the therapeutic relationship.

In their next session, the therapist was able to open a successful dialogue with Lorraine about her feelings of fear and loss related to her deteriorating health and independence. The therapist encouraged Lorraine to be upset with her for missing their appointment, and to also consider Lorraine's comment that she "was worried about" her therapist. Lorraine recognized that her initial worry about her therapist represented her own worries about ending treatment because of her own failing health. In response to this revelation, Lorraine remarked that it was a relief to talk about "growing old and fat and unfashionable." She observed that her friends and relatives referred to her as the "always young, fun one" who was never encouraged to discuss her own problems or fears. No one seemed to want to hear about her most recent visit to the eye doctor; they would rather hear stories about the cruise she took last month or the new earrings she just bought. Lorraine's therapist provided her with a unique opportunity to discuss her thoughts and fears about aging, and to devise ways to deal with the resistance to aging she encountered within her own peer group. When Lorraine later moved to a nursing home unit during the following year, her therapist also felt more prepared and accepting of this change, and the two were able to continue their sessions in this different setting.

Additional Reactions

When working with an elderly patient for which sexual issues become the focus of treatment, an even greater variety of feelings can ensue (see Apfel, Fox, Isberg, & Levine, 1984). These reactions are quite similar to those experienced when working with sexually sensitive issues with younger patients, but these feelings may be magnified by the unusualness of the situation for the therapist. Pervasive societal beliefs that elderly sexuality is inappropriate or impossible also lend themselves to stronger and more ambivalent reactions. Typical countertransference reactions to elderly patients whose cases involve sexual issues often include:

- Embarrassment
- Disgust, with subsequent feelings of shame and guilt about the initial feelings of disgust
- Titillation and voyeuristic tendencies
- Competitiveness
- Sexual attraction
- Denial of sexual attraction
- Disorientation
- Intrusive thoughts of parents or grandparents
- Acute awareness of body image

Many therapists are shocked when they find themselves attracted to an elderly patient. Poggi and Berland (1985) provide one of the few discussions of this in the literature. They describe group therapists' positive reactions to an attractive woman in her 70s. They further note that since they have been involved in such work for more than 6 years, this probably was a novel experience for them because their sexual feelings for other attractive, older patients were categorically repressed and denied. Most clinicians find such sexual attraction to their older patients unsettling and sometimes, even alarming. Often, once a practitioner realizes that this experience is certainly within the normal range of experience, anxiety about this reaction subsides and it becomes easier to interpret the basis of the attraction.

Allen

As with younger patients, feelings of sexual attraction often provide useful, diagnostic information. Allen was a soldier during World War II. Before he went off to war, he was married and had two children. After his return from Europe, things began to change for Allen. His marriage dissolved, and he began to drink heavily. As he aged, he divorced his first wife, married another woman, divorced this second wife, became estranged from his children, and then married for the third time. By the time he was 68, he was in the hospital for a bilateral, above-the-knee amputation. Allen had developed diabetes, and between his diabetes, substance abuse, and poor attention to medical care, both of his legs had to be amputated. Soon after this traumatic event, Allen suffered a stroke in which he lost movement on his left side. Since he was left-handed, he struggled to even feed himself. His wife, who lived more than 40 minutes away from the hospital, found it difficult to take three different bus and train lines to visit him very often.

When his therapist first met Allen, she could not help but be shocked by his appearance. Allen appeared to be a thin man, even when he was in good physical shape. His face was pale and gaunt, and what little hair he had left was thin and pure white. He always lay under covers, propped up by some pillows. The thin blankets left nothing to the imagination; Allen's body appeared to be a short stump, and his left arm hung limp at his side. His therapist felt anxious and uncomfortable when she thought about his missing limbs and felt helpless thinking about being in his position. Allen was quite depressed, and expressed wishes to hang himself with the phone cord by his bed. He cried when all of the cords were moved away from the reach of his right hand.

Despite the depth of his depression, Allen was a willing and active participant in therapy. He spoke at length about his service in the war, and about his one grandson who lived in London and worked as a journalist. Allen also lamented that all he did all day was watch TV, and that it was like watching everyone else through a big window. No one could see him or hear him on his side. Although it was tempting to fall into Allen's passive-dependent stance, his therapist helped Allen learn to strike up conversation with his nurses, to ask to be moved outside during the day in a karol chair, and to have special remote controls and forks provided for him so that he could feed himself and change the channels easily on his own television. Within a few months, he denied any suicidal ideation and focused on renewing his relationship with his children and grandson. He was not yet able to cope with the ambivalent nature of the relationship with his third wife, however.

Suddenly, his therapist began to notice things about Allen that she had not noticed before. She noticed his bright green eyes, the colors used in the tattoos on his upper arms, and his ability to joke with the nursing staff. One day, Allen asked her to look at a card that his daughter sent to him, and his hand brushed against her as he clumsily handed her the card. For a brief moment, his therapist noticed the warmth of his hand, and for a moment felt physically attracted to Allen. Once the moment had passed, his therapist felt baffled and somewhat bemused. While she previously felt very protective and maternal toward her patient (and had worked hard not to act on those feelings), she began to regard him with more respect and interest once she was able to rid herself of feeling embarrassed about the exchange.

Deciding to investigate this countertransferential reaction further, Allen's therapist decided to broach the subject of sexuality and Allen's relationship to his wife. Allen responded that he had not had sex with his wife since his legs were amputated. He added, "These nurses are wonderful to me and everything, but there are times when I wish I didn't have that tube (catheter) stuck up my there [in my penis]. I guess I'm more used to it now." Allen added that while he did not think he would ever have sex again, "the whole thing," he still wished his wife would come to visit him and sit with him in bed, hold his hand, or just kiss him. While he previously expressed remorse and sadness about his condition, and felt that his wife had every reason to feel revolted by him, he began to assert his own needs and wants and to express anger toward her. "In sickness and health, my ass.... Even my own kids are starting to call me and visit me. What about her?"

Apparently, the therapist's attraction to Allen represented an unconscious fulfillment of his desire to be seen as attractive by another member of the opposite sex, and a recognition on the part of his therapist that Allen was ready for more insight oriented work and a greater sense of entitlement. Allen's therapist also gained insight into the relationship between sex, power, and self-esteem. This relationship can be particularly salient for an older adult who feels that his or her body, as well as body image, is distorted or damaged.

Transference

Just as it is vital that clinicians evaluate their own emotional reactions to their elderly patients, elderly patients often have strong conscious and unconscious emotional responses to their typically younger therapists. Because transference is often regarded as an unconscious process, it is important to note that an elderly person who has a therapist 45 years his or her junior may still manifest a transference in which the elderly patient regards the younger therapist as a maternal figure. The age difference between therapist and patient initially may prevent therapists from considering the wide range of transference configurations available in their interaction. In sum, clinicians must remember that transference is not age or reality based; patients and therapists of any age combination can provide the backdrop for any number of transferential interactions.

Eroticized Transference

A particularly difficult transference reaction for clinicians to manage both personally and professionally is that of an eroticized transference. Patients may make blatant or subtle sexualized comments toward the therapist, or may act out sexual urges in the form of inappropriate attempts to touch their therapist, to sit too close to them, or to give suggestive gifts. Other patients may make inappropriate statements pertaining directly to sexual attributes of the therapist or to wishes for sexual liaisons. Although it is more common for female patients to develop eroticized transferences to their male therapists, male patients also have been reported to develop such eroticized transferences to their female therapists (Lester, 1985). Regardless of the sex of the patient or therapist, these interactions often are among the most disturbing events cited by both novice and experienced therapists. However, these challenges in therapy can lead to the uncovering of significant conflicts and to beneficial changes in the therapeutic relationship and the patient's life. As with younger patients, such sexualized interactions directed by the patient toward the therapist often mask deep-seated patient issues involving interpersonal power, boundary problems, a resistance to change (Blum, 1973; Rappaport, 1956), and both fears of and needs for intimacy (Peterson, Levin, & Zweig, 1989) in their own relationships.

Mario

Mario, a 67-year-old retired husband of 43 years and father of three, sought treatment for major depression. He had become so depressed that he lay in bed for most of the day, and it took significant effort on the part of his wife to get him out of bed to eat and shower. Mario remarked that he knew he needed treatment when he realized that for the first time, he could not stand to hear his grandchildren running and playing through the house. His wife also became very frustrated that her husband was no longer interested in attending social functions or going out to restaurants with friends, and insisted that he seek treatment. Mario had always assumed the role of provider, protector, and entertainer. He lamented that before he became depressed, he was "always the center of the party" and that he was always the one to make the toast or command an audience for an impromptu speech. Mario's depression emerged at approximately the same time he retired from his position as head salesman at a local construction company. His depression worsened when he learned that his son was going to declare bankruptcy; Mario was despondent that he did not have the money to get his son out of financial trouble.

During the course of his treatment, Mario worked hard to schedule interesting activities for himself and to become educated about depression. He became less frightened that any negative feeling would grow into an overwhelming, incapacitating experience of depression. He had begun to enjoy his grandchildren and had successfully ventured out on a few evenings for dinners with his wife and other couples. He also had begun to accept that his son had made some bad financial decisions, and that he did not have to feel guilty about not having the money to prevent his son from filing for bankruptcy. Once his depression had begun to lift, Mario began to spend more time in treatment on the conflicted relationship he had with his wife (i.e., women).

A discussion of his marriage revealed that Mario maintained very traditional sex roles. He expected that his wife cook, clean, and take care of the grandchildren whenever they came to visit. He also expressed anger and concern that his youngest daughter was working outside of the home. When asked what about her job made him so angry, he said that if she were any kind of self-respecting woman and mother, she would stay at home to care for her children and let her husband be the breadwinner in the family. When asked what it was like for him to have a female therapist, who obviously worked outside of the home and who was even a bit younger than his own daughter, Mario responded, "It doesn't matter because you are a professional, and you are here to help me. How you decide to spend your personal time is not up to me."

When his therapist added that it sometimes can be difficult for people to work closely with someone who has different values than you have, Mario retorted, "Well, Doc, it's OK with me. You are helping me out. You have a Ph.D. That is a special deal, for a man or a woman. I don't mind, really." Mario went on further to discuss that he had known one other Ph.D. in his life, and she was "a terrific lady" who was his boss for the last 15 years. He became resistant to discussing the issue further, either from the perspective of sex roles, his own career expectations, or his own competitiveness. Mario's therapist decided that at least she was able to broach the issue even if he were not prepared to discuss it at that particular time.

The next week, Mario canceled his session without notice. The following week, he presented his therapist with a bottle of cheap perfume. (His therapist's policy on gifts was that she would take gifts only if they were inexpensive, and only on the condition that her patient was willing to process the interaction.) Mario's therapist attempted to hide her discomfort and thanked him for the gift. She also asked Mario if he were comfortable discussing it because it could be helpful to him in his therapy, in terms of better understanding their relationship and his relationship with other people in his life. Although Mario had been open to such self-exploration previously, he replied, "But, I don't understand. It's only a gift I got at a wholesale price from my nephew. He's got a job at [a store] and always had a big discount, you know." He mentioned that if his therapist were a man, he would have selected a "man's gift," like a wallet or a coupon toward new tires on a car. Mario denied that the choice of perfume was meaningful, or that his gift could be related to anything that had happened in a prior session, such as mixed feelings over his therapist's credentials, sex, and values.

During the next week's session, Mario focused on his relationship with his old boss, "the other lady with the Ph.D." He mentioned that "even though she was a woman," she could get along with any man, and tell any joke. She also appeared to guide Mario's rise through the ranks before he moved to his current position at a different branch of the company. He began to tell a graphic story about a friend of his who sold "big brassieres." Mario gave his therapist a wink and said, "You ladies know all about them, right, Doc?" Toward the end of the session, Mario's therapist coughed (she had a cold) and Mario retorted, "Hey, Doc, I know CPR. Do you think you need some mouth to mouth?" Mario's therapist began to feel embarrassed and uncomfortable by this inappropriate attention and innuendo. When she attempted to process these points with Mario, and asked him how he thought she might respond to those questions, he changed the subject or denied what he had said.

When the session had concluded, Mario's therapist's response to his inappropriate sexual comments began to change from feelings of discomfort and anxiety to feelings of anger and oppression. She recognized that these advances were not motivated by a desire for intimacy, but were motivated by Mario's conscious or unconscious desire to assert control through the use of sexual domination. He did not have a wish to "save her" from a coughing spell, but instead desired to, in effect, castrate her with his own sexual innuendo in order to overwhelm her and make her feel less like a professional. During the following session, Mario's therapist informed him that it was an important part of his treatment that they discuss, as openly as they could, what had happened during the previous week. Mario's therapist also suggested that if they could understand what was happening between the two of them, it might give Mario some insight into the problems he was having in his own marriage and in his feelings toward his prior boss.

Mario sat quietly for a moment and agreed to attempt to talk about what had happened. He said that he never had an affair with his old boss, but that "it sure had been tempting." He was confused but titillated and excited by his old boss's ability to move easily among both men and women. Mario recounted a time in which he drove her to a formal dinner party, and she wore a beaded gown that fit her "just right in all the right places." He found it hard to believe that someone who could "swear a blue streak with the rest of us" could look that way in a dress. He felt proud to be singled out as her special assistant; she made sure that he was placed on the best jobs with the best overtime rates and chances for advancement.

When asked if he ever wanted to give his boss CPR or mouth-to-mouth, he said emphatically that their relationship was never sexual. However, he added that once or twice, when he drove her to business dinners, she often would ask him to come inside the ladies' room and make sure that no one would come inside while she was changing. When asked how she looked while she was changing, Mario responded, "Oh, she knew and I knew that I would keep my eyes on the door while she was in there changing." Only then did Mario acknowledge that he might have had mixed feelings about his boss. He also was able to see that while unusual requests played into his traditional expectations about sex roles and his desire to protect her and assert his sexuality with her, they were anything but professional. She was, in fact, coming on to him the way he typically imagined a man would come on to a woman.

Mario also recognized that his primary experience with professional women was with this woman, who was very different than his wife, his mother, his friends' wives, and his daughter. His boss, the woman with the Ph.D., seemed to marry power with sex. When asked if his boss reminded him of anyone, he responded sheepishly that he had placed a lot of emphasis on the fact that his therapist had a Ph.D. With more gentle questioning, he also admitted that, just like with his boss, he had thought about what it would be like to go on a date, or to go out to dinner. At this point, his therapist had to take a moment to collect herself, and to put aside her discomfort at discussing this topic herself. Mario's therapist reinforced that while their relationship was professional, and would always remain professional, discussing such feelings could be important in helping him understand how he relates to woman in general, and to his wife in particular. Mario said that since it "was OK just to talk about it, then," he would enjoy going out to dinner with his therapist, talking about interesting things, and "showing her off" to his friends. He added quickly, "I wouldn't really even think about having sex with you, I mean, at least on the first few dates. Talking is really important to me." Mario realized that his feelings toward his therapist (which he now said had faded quickly since they talked about them) mirrored those that he had thought about his old boss, but had never really allowed himself to think about. He also recalled that the first Christmas after his boss had asked him to "watch out for her" in the ladies' room, he gave her a small gift of perfume at the office party.

Now that Mario recognized his underlying feelings of sexual attraction for his old boss, coupled with his feelings of impotence about being her subordinate, his eroticized transference toward his therapist dissipated quickly and allowed for a previously buried conflict to surface in its place. Mario was now able to compare his feelings for his old boss and his wife, and process his own ambivalence about having a woman who could both excite him sexually and be in a position of power at the same time. Mario traditionally viewed his wife as his subordinate, and recognized that he could still feel aroused by her. He also recognized that he had fallen victim to the traditional "Madonna/whore conflict" (although his therapist did not discuss this conflict in these specific terms) in which he viewed powerful, freewheeling women such as his boss as sexual beings, and he viewed subordinate, material women such as his wife as nonsexual beings. The enactment of an erotic transference to his female therapist also is suggestive of wishes to merge with a "vengeful, overpowering, phallic mother" (p. 284) as manifested via issues of dominance and submission (Lester, 1985).

As the transference was interpreted and dispelled, Mario also felt less guilty about his romantic feelings for his boss because he learned that she actively contributed to the sexualized nature of their relationship. He also was reassured when his therapist pointed out that even in such enticing situations, Mario placed his faithfulness to his wife, his marriage, and his family first in his life; he could experience a variety of feelings without acting on them. Toward the end of his therapy, Mario's depression faded significantly, and he noted that he had begun to enjoy his wife's company more, both in and out of the bedroom. He began to enjoy his retirement more, and became intrigued by the fact that his wife was somewhat like the new "boss" of domestic chores at home. He began to learn to untie his relationship between sex and control, and understand that both he and his wife could be powerful and sexual.

June

June was an 83-year-old white, divorced woman who lived in a nursing home. She had been married and divorced twice, and had no children. She lost her brother and two sisters to cancer 5 years previously. Her only family contact was with a nephew who lived in another state. He visited once in the last 5 years, and would only occasionally telephone June on major holidays. Essentially, June had no family or friends to visit her. She suffered from bipolar disorder, and during her manic periods she could become bitter and cruel to others. Most of her friends appeared to shy away from her once they were aware of what she was capable of doing and saying. June also had physical problems that made it rare for her to get out of bed, and she needed a wheelchair to move around the home.

June was a willing participant in psychotherapy. She had been stabilized on her medication for about a year, and was able to engage in meaningful conversation with some degree of introspection. Most of her treatment revolved around accepting her physical limitations and making attempts to develop friendships within the nursing home. June often felt that the other residents were "beneath" her since they suffered from some cognitive impairments. Other residents' physical deterioration represented an unpleasant reflection of her own narcissistic injury, and she felt uneasy in their presence.

Knowing her history of poor interpersonal relations, even when she was younger and physically healthy, her therapist had guarded expectations about June's ability to have intimate peer relationships. During her treatment, June decided to pursue craft classes and music hours. Her mood brightened and she began to eat in the community dining room instead of her room. (She often ate by herself, but at least made the effort to socialize.) June also began to remark to her therapist about a "wonderful young man who comes to visit." Her therapist was surprised to learn that this visitor was not her nephew, but a janitorial aid who stopped in to talk to June during his night shift. He did not appear to be motivated by money or other favors (June was practically indigent), and visited her at least once a week. June enjoyed these visits very much, and said that it was nice to have someone who was smart enough to play cards with her and to talk about things she heard on the news.

Approximately a month later, June became insolent and angry. She threw a food tray at a staff member and refused to come out of her room for hours at a time. When her therapist asked her what was going on, she said that her special friend had not been to visit for a few days. When asked if he might be sick or on vacation, she muttered, "Oh, I think I know what happened." Apparently, June had begun to "joke around" with her visitor. She said she thought it was funny that she began to refer to him as her "boyfriend," and she teased him about his nice eyes and dark hair. She also said that she told him that if she were his age, "I wouldn't let you get past my bedroom." She also admitted that the last time she saw him, she reached over and pinched him on the waist. Without a formal or professional relationship, this kindly visitor probably became overwhelmed by such sexualized responses from an elderly, physically disabled woman, and simply stopped coming by to visit. Her violation of his personal, physical boundaries appeared to be the most disturbing episode. Perhaps understandably, the eroticized transference she projected onto this young man simply was too much for him to tolerate.

June's therapist was sure to check on her mental status; she was not becoming manic nor did she deviate from taking her psychotropic medication. Apparently, June's emerging feelings of intimacy with this visitor and her therapist were too threatening; she had little experience with true intimacy and her underlying personality issues prevented her from getting close to others in the past. To continue in this trend, she found some way to become too loathsome for her visitor to tolerate. He was accepting of her age and her physical disability; it is as though she had to generate some other means to thwart his friendship. June's therapist was only somewhat successful in guiding her in processing her actions. June maintained that "I'm no spring chicken, but I still find young men very attractive." She used her socially appropriate desires to promote herself as sexual in old age as a foil for socially inappropriate behaviors with an unrequiting, younger adult. June's eroticized transference to this visitor represented an attempt to use sex in order to thwart genuine, emotional intimacy.

Guides to Managing the Transference

The first step in managing such a transference, particularly an eroticized transference, is to recognize that it is diagnostic, and an indicator that either consciously or unconsciously, enough trust and rapport has been established in the therapeutic relationship to allow it to enfold (Peterson et al., 1989). The second step is for the therapist to accept that any emotional reaction to such a transference, whether it is anger, embarrassment, arousal, confusion, oppression, pleasure, anxiety, or any other emotion, is entirely normal. In short, clinicians must be prepared for an onslaught of powerful and often disconcerting feelings. Therapists also must remember that while it is normal to experience any of these emotions, they must proceed carefully in order to avoid acting on them.

The third step in managing the transference is often the most difficult for clinicians. The patient's fantasies about the therapist must be discussed at length, in order for appropriate reality testing to take place (Rappaport, 1956). Patients should be encouraged to recognize that this sexualized pattern of relating that they have created with their therapist parallels an important relationship or conflict in their own lives. In discussing such an eroticized transference, both patients and clinicians are reassured by clear, unambiguous messages that the relationship between them is, always will be, and must always remain purely professional. Talking about feelings will always remain separate from acting on them in the therapeutic relationship, and the therapist is well prepared to handle any feelings that the patient brings to the session (also see Rappaport, 1956). Patients are often comforted by such demonstrative statements that appropriate boundaries will be maintained, and that firm limits are in place for what is considered safe, acceptable behavior.

Ultimately, patients recognize that sexual interactions do not necessarily arise from benevolent, loving feelings; they may indeed underlie aggressive, hostile feelings or intentions (Blum, 1973; Lester, 1985; Rappaport, 1956). When the therapist can maintain neutrality and objectivity, patients begin to learn that their illusions within the therapeutic relationship reflect real, but often alterable conflicts within their own interpersonal relationships. As difficult as it is for therapists to manage these eroticized transferences, they often provide one of the best means of assessing our patients' underlying character structure and core conflicts.

## SUMMARY

Attitudes toward elderly sexuality play a powerful and important role in the sexual identity and expression of older adults. The attitudes maintained by society at large, elderly adults themselves, and the health care providers who treat them are equally important items for exploration. Self-report measures such as the attitude subscale of the ASKAS (White, 1982) can be used to initiate discussion of often undisclosed thoughts and feelings. The therapeutic relationship also is ripe with powerful countertransference and transference issues. Clinicians must be aware of their own, potentially sexualized feelings toward their elderly patients, and also be aware of the presence of any sexualized attitudes directed at them by their patients.

Although one of the most difficult subjects to broach, an analysis of such transference and countertransference can provide some of the most valuable information regarding an elderly patients' attitudes toward sexuality, their sense of intrinsic value, sex role conflicts, and difficulties with or needs for intimacy. As in our work with younger patients, having a variety of countertransferential feelings is acceptable and typically unavoidable. It is how we decide to process and act on these feelings that makes the therapeutic relationship so beneficial. Elderly adults who seek treatment for sexual issues, or for whom sexual issues emerge in treatment, often need reassurance from their health care provider that talking about any feeling in relation to this topic is welcomed and permitted. Because society provides a closed door in relation to elderly sexuality, we as clinicians must ensure that we offer the proverbial, open door to issues of elderly sexuality. We have the unique opportunity to provide a corrective educational and emotional experience for our elderly patients.

# 4

# Elderly Sexuality
# within an Institutional Context

*Nursing home staff members have identified residents' inappropriate sexual behaviors as among some of the most disturbing events that they experience on the job, and as a significant source of work-related stress.*

Many people regard nursing homes as "god's waiting room" or a place for elderly people to die. Many clinicians report having an aversion to working with institutionalized older adults, for a variety of reasons. Clinicians have described the following barriers to their involvement with patients in nursing home care settings:

- Confusion regarding the intersection among medical problems, medical treatment, and psychiatric care
- Discomfort with the sights and smells inherent in a long term care facility
- Problems in navigating cryptic administrative and policy issues
- Antagonistic relationships between staff psychiatrists, internists, and nursing personnel
- Expectations that patients have no hope for improvement
- Fears of becoming emotionally attached to patients who soon may die
- Low levels of reimbursement from federally and state funded insurance plans such as Medicare and Medicaid
- Difficulties in filling out the paperwork for such insurance plans and subsequent delays in receiving payment

It is notable that the vast majority of clinicians do not even cite concerns regarding the expression of elderly sexuality as a deterrent to working in an institutional setting. Instead, concerns about institutionalized sexuality appear to be superseded by feelings and fears of aging, hopelessness, and inevitable decline. Consistent with negative societal expectations, thoughts of elderly sexuality within an institution appear generally to be an afterthought, or even an implausibility.

For those who do work closely with institutionalized elderly adults, however, nursing home staff members—psychologists, psychiatrists, internists, nutritionists, social workers, nurses, nursing aides, and occupational and physical therapists—find that their work with infirm elderly patients is among both the most demanding and rewarding work that they have ever performed. They learn that elderly adults do have outlets for growth and change, and they often come to accept the physical decline that accompanies their patients' care. However, these same staff members also report that incidents regarding elderly sexuality are more common than uncommon in their workday, and that they find them among the most disturbing "problem behaviors" that they encounter (Wallace, 1992).

The range of sexual behaviors manifested by elderly residents in nursing homes and other institutions varies widely. The expression of sexual feelings and desires may range from more sublime expressions such as taking evening walks, giving a massage, and holding hands to more overt expressions such as hugging, kissing, petting, fondling, and intercourse. Along this continuum of behaviors, it is notable that these more overt expressions of sexuality, in which personal boundaries are traversed, typically require an element of privacy, something in short supply in many institutional settings. Sexual activity among institutionalized elderly adults also may be characterized by the actual number of residents involved. In the case of fulfilling sexual desires through special attention to grooming or through masturbation, such sexual expression may be solitary. In contrast, behaviors such as kissing, fondling, petting, sexual intercourse, and clearly inappropriate behaviors such as voyeurism and exhibitionism necessarily involve two or more parties. When such sexual behavior involves two or more elderly residents, important questions must be addressed regarding the consensual nature of the interaction and the cognitive status of the parties involved.

In sum, sexual expression among institutionalized elderly is multifaceted and presents itself in a variety of contexts. A number of dimensions can be evaluated including the individual or collective nature of the interaction, the extent to which body boundaries are traversed, the need and availability of privacy, and the competency of the elderly residents. It becomes vital for staff members to ascertain whether these patients' sexual behaviors are truly problematic and inappropriate, or whether otherwise well-intentioned staff members are introducing their own stereotypes and prejudices on their elderly charges.

## A SELF-TEST FOR ATTITUDES

As health care providers, we would like to regard our own attitudes toward elderly sexuality as very different from the typically negative, global attitudes espoused by mainstream society. However, it often is difficult to articulate, much less begin to appraise, one's own attitudes toward elderly sexuality. When asked to consider their own attitudes toward elderly sexuality, many practitioners and older adults alike have commented simply, "Well … I never really thought about it before." The attitude section of the ASKAS (White, 1982) provides us with a self-report measure that easily allows clinicians, health care providers, adult children of older adults, and older adults themselves to assess their attitudes toward elderly sexuality, particularly within the context of an institutional setting. It is comprised of 26 items that can be answered using a seven-point Likert scale. The scale also can be useful in generating discussion about potentially sensitive sexual issues among older adults, older adult couples, and among older adults and their family members. A number of topics are addressed including institutional sexuality, sexual mores, and masturbation. The attitude scale items from the ASKAS are presented below. Persons formally taking the test are instructed to use the following scale to evaluate each question:

| 1 | 2 | 3 | 4 | 5 | 6 | 7 |
|---|---|---|---|---|---|---|
| Disagree | | | | | | Agree |

Otherwise, persons taking the subtest are simply advised to think about each question, and consider their initial reaction.

1. Elderly people have little interest in sexuality (elderly or aged = 65+ years of age).
2. An aged person who shows sexual interest brings disgrace to himself or herself.
3. Institutions, such as nursing homes, ought not to encourage or support sexual activity of any sort in its residences.
4. Male and female residents of nursing homes ought to live on separate floors or separate wings of the nursing home.
5. Nursing homes have no obligation to provide adequate privacy for residents who desire to be alone, either by themselves or as a couple.
6. As one becomes older (say past 65) interest in sexuality inevitably disappears.

For items 7–9: If a relative of mine, living in a nursing home, were to have a sexual relationship with another resident I would ...

7. Complain to the management.
8. Move my relative from this institution.
9. Stay out of it as it is not my concern.
10. If I knew that a particular nursing home permitted and supported sexual activity in residents who desired it, I would not place a relative in that nursing home.
11. It is immoral for older persons to engage in recreational sex.
12. I would like to know more about the changes in sexual functioning in older years.
13. I feel I know all I need to know about sexuality in the aged.
14. I would complain to the management if I knew of sexual activity between any residents of a nursing home.
15. I would support sex education courses for aged residents of nursing homes.
16. I would support sex education courses for the staff of nursing homes.

17. Masturbation is an acceptable sexual activity for older males.
18. Masturbation is an acceptable sexual activity for older females.
19. Institutions such as nursing homes ought to provide large enough beds for couples who desire to sleep together.
20. Staff of nursing homes ought to be trained or educated with regard to sexuality in the aged and disabled.
21. Residents of nursing homes ought not to engage in sexual activity of any sort.
22. Institutions such as nursing homes should provide opportunities for the social interaction of men and women.
23. Masturbation is harmful and ought to be avoided.
24. Institutions such as nursing homes should provide privacy to allow residents to engage in sexual behavior without fear of intrusion or observation.
25. If a family member objects to a widowed relative engaging in sexual relations with another resident of a nursing home, it is the obligation of the management and staff to make certain that such sexual activity is prevented.
26. Sexual relations outside the context of marriage are always wrong.

A series of additional attitudinal questions have been employed in conjunction with the attitude subscale of the ASKAS (Hillman & Stricker, 1996). These were designed to spur additional interest and conversation among its test takers. These few, additional items are to be addressed with the seven-point Likert scale employed by the ASKAS.

27. If I found out that an elderly relative of mine were engaging in sexual activity, I would be delighted.
28. It is easy for me to imagine elderly couples in loving, romantic sexual relationships.
29. Masturbation among elderly people without partners should be encouraged, so that they have a sexual outlet.
30. Sexuality is a wonderful thing to express at any age.
31. Physicians should talk to elderly people about sexual relations on a regular basis.
32. I would feel very comfortable having a conversation about elderly sexuality.

## ATTITUDES AMONG HEALTH CARE PROVIDERS

### Related Research Findings

The attitude subscale of the ASKAS has provided the brunt of the empirical data available regarding individuals' attitudes toward elderly sexuality. General research findings suggest that health care providers possess more permissive than restrictive attitudes toward elderly sexuality (Damrosch, 1984; Damrosch & Fischman, 1985; Glass, Mustian, & Carter, 1986; Glass & Webb, 1995; White &

Catania, 1982). However, individual case studies about institutionalized patients' "problem behaviors" and individual attitude items addressing more specific behaviors such as masturbation among elderly patients (Damrosch, 1984; Hillman & Stricker, 1996; Poggi & Berland, 1985; Szasz, 1983) have been found to elicit significantly more guarded and negative responses (Wallace, 1992). It is as though practitioners are responding to demands for political correctness, or are intending to profess more positive attitudes until they are forced to deal with specific incidents that evoke anxiety and other unpleasant feelings within the context of the therapeutic relationship.

It is one thing to talk abstractly about an elderly person's sexual behavior, and quite another to speak at length, in detail, with an institutionalized elderly woman who wants to learn how to masturbate to orgasm, or to walk into a patient's room (after first knocking and obtaining permission) to find the roommate with advanced Alzheimer's disease masturbating openly. Nursing home staff members also may cope with such incidents in a variety of ways, both professional and unprofessional. It often becomes the role of the clinician to guide other staff members in their management of such situations. Psychologists in nursing homes often find that they provide as much "treatment" and support for staff members as for patients when issues of elderly sexuality are involved.

## Richard

Richard was an 81-year-old man living in a nursing home. He suffered from Alzheimer's dementia, and was in the final stages of the illness. Richard required assistance in feeding, dressing, bathing, and toileting himself. He was no longer able to speak or to move easily about the unit. Richard's weight had dwindled to nearly 110 pounds, though he stood more than 6 feet tall. Although he did not receive individual psychotherapy because of his severely impaired mental status, the unit psychologist encouraged all staff members to actively involve Richard in occupational, music, and pet therapy. When engaged directly in such activities, Richard displayed a gentle character, and would sometimes smile and make gurgling noises.

When not engaged in planned activities, Richard spent most of his time during the day in the third floor lounge. He often was placed in a karol chair to help maintain his posture. The staff members took care to have him sit next to other gentlemen who were in a similar state. Even though they could not talk to each other, they would sometimes look at each other, reach out to tap each other's arms, and smile. The staff reported that Richard was an easygoing man who was easy to provide care for. He was widowed, and his four children lived out of state. He had no visitors. Although the staff psychologist did not know Richard well, she was well aware of his status and she conducted periodic assessments with him.

When walking through the unit to have a therapy session with a patient who was bed bound, the psychologist heard an announcement over the public announcement system, "We have a naked man here in the lounge and we need help.... Mr. N. is taking his pants off. [laughter] We need a nursing assistant right now!" The psychologist rounded the corner in time to see the unit receptionist buckled over in laughter, two of the nurses rushing to Richard's aid, and one of the occupational therapists shading his eyes and walking back to his office. Richard was standing up in front of his karol chair, with his pajama bottoms around his knees. (He was not wearing any underwear.) Richard was shaking from the effort of supporting himself, and there was concern that he would fall. The psychologist grabbed the microphone from the receptionist to stop her from broadcasting over the public address system. Within a few minutes, Richard was helped back into his pants, and was taken to the bathroom to see if he needed to void.

Although Richard appeared to be unscathed from this incident, a number of patients and staff members were noticeably disturbed. The receptionist was saying loudly enough for other patients in the hallways and in adjacent rooms to hear, "I didn't want to see Richard's thing! Put that nasty thing away. He is one wrinkly, old dude.... Oh, my God! That was so disgusting." Patients who were moving about the unit appeared embarrassed to see another patient's genitals. Some seemed to laugh off the incident, while others hung their heads and slowly walked away or to their rooms. The primary concern for the psychologist was that the other, observant patients were thinking that if they were to lose control of their faculties, would they be treated with such disrespect and disdain by the people whom they depended on to care for them? Regarding the patients' concerns, the psychologist held a support group (e.g., Hodson & Skeen, 1994) a few days later in which issues of privacy, sexuality, and expectations for care were discussed. Individual patients also were approached after the incident to ask them about what they saw and how they interpreted both Richard's behavior and the staff members' responses to it.

After this incident was rectified and documented, the psychologist was able to speak informally with the receptionist and members of the nursing staff who were present. The receptionist was informed gently but directly that it is essential that patients are never laughed at or humiliated, particularly in front of other patients. The receptionist also was provided with emotional support, and was able to admit that she was so shocked and upset about seeing this elderly man naked that her first reaction was to laugh and make a joke out of it. She seemed to accept that although humor is a good way to dispel tension and discomfort, it must never be expressed openly at a patient's expense. The receptionist was helped to devise a plan that if such an event were to happen again, she would immediately, and privately, seek out the assistance of a trained nurse or other staff member involved in primary care. The psychologist and nursing staff also were able to counsel the receptionist that she could expect to see more patient nudity, even if that was not in her job description. In sum, the use of a team approach led to the most effective resolution of a potentially serious problem.

Gregory

Gregory was a 71-year-old single man who lived in and out of a nursing home for rehabilitative needs after several heart surgeries and fractures from falls. He was moderately depressed and also presented with dependent personality disorder. Gregory had been active in hand-to-hand combat during World War II, and lamented that he was now forced to use a walker to get around. He also was no longer allowed to drive because of his glaucoma and slowed reflexes. Despite these physical limitations and insults to his previous independence, Gregory faithfully attended a day hospital program on the nursing home grounds. He enjoyed talking and joking with the other patients and learned how to paint and to work with ceramics. He also participated in psychotherapy on a weekly basis in order to help him cope with the changes in his physical health and his subsequent depression.

During therapy, Gregory liked to display his newest works of art. He often made things for other patients in the nursing home who "couldn't get around as well as [he could]." Soon, however, he began to make more and more pieces for a woman whom he was dating. He reluctantly admitted to his therapist that even though he had his own apartment when he was not required to stay at the nursing home for care, he often spent the nights and weekends with his "lady friend" at her own home. He seemed relieved to learn that the psychologist had no intention of judging his behavior, but was more interested in helping him decide how he felt about his relationship with this woman. Gregory disclosed that he was concerned that his girlfriend would abandon him in favor of another man who was more physically fit. He said that even though the physician told him it was OK for him to have intercourse with her, he sometimes felt scared that he would suffer another heart attack. He also found it difficult to discuss these concerns with his girlfriend directly.

Gregory's paranoia grew when he mentioned to his psychologist that he tried to call his girlfriend a few times a day, just to find out what she was doing. His girlfriend appeared to grow tired of this oppressive observation, and told Gregory that she would only talk to him in the evenings; she had errands to run and friends to visit during the day. Gregory also revealed that he gave more than half of his pension check to his girlfriend, even when he was unsure if she were being faithful to him. Things began to escalate quickly when Gregory hit another patient at the nursing home. When Gregory was waiting for an elevator, a wheelchair bound patient with dementia ran into his injured leg. Gregory's immediate response was to strike out and hit the patient in the wheelchair with his cane. A nurse on duty documented the incident, and Gregory was asked to appear before the treatment team for a meeting to discuss his behavior.

During this treatment team meeting in which Gregory was asked to evaluate his assaultive behavior, the unit psychologist elicited more information from Gregory that he was becoming increasingly paranoid that his girlfriend didn't love him anymore. He became obsessed that she might be having an affair with another man. He was upset that they had planned a weekend trip to the mountains (she was going to pick him up and drive them to the cottage), and that his girlfriend had canceled at the last minute. When Gregory asked her why she didn't want to go, she responded curtly that she was going on vacation, but that she was going to go "with a friend" instead. Gregory was devastated when his girlfriend would not answer his question, "So is it a male or female friend?" It also was unclear to the treatment team members whether his girlfriend (who also appeared to have her own mental health problems) was invested in maintaining their relationship or not. The treatment team informed Gregory that while it was understandable he was upset, such abusive behavior toward other patients was unacceptable. He was encouraged to vent his feelings through his therapy and through his art.

When discussing the issue with the treatment team privately, Gregory's psychologist brought up the difficulties he was having with issues of power, sex, and masculinity and the potential benefits of couples counseling. Other members of the treatment team seemed nonplussed, and remarked that he was lucky to have a girlfriend of any variety at this point in his life. Others remarked that since he was not married, couple's counseling might not be effective. Another team member would not even refer to this woman as Gregory's girlfriend; she insisted on referring to her as his *paramour*. It was as though labeling her as "his girlfriend" would elicit concerns and issues that were too realistic and personal. The term *paramour* itself seems to carry additional, negative implications of antiquated times, artificial formality devoid of intimacy, and "dirty" or improper sex with a concubine or philanderer.

When asked about the implications directly, many staff members avoided the topic and remarked that they were simply concerned for Gregory's health; if he had a heart attack and was using a walker, how could he possibly have a sexual relationship? Despite assurances from the team physician that Gregory could engage in sexual activity, many team members appeared unconvinced. Quite simply, the treatment team members' prejudices and fears were projected onto Gregory. It took a substantial amount of group work for many of the team members to acknowledge their own feelings, and to legitimize those of Gregory. One of the team members remained unconvinced that this patient had "sufficient reason" to be so upset. Ultimately, Gregory's girlfriend broke off ties with him, and he was able to receive support from the majority of the team members as he mourned his loss. It had become clear that Gregory was not inappropriately paranoid; his girlfriend admitted to seeing another man while he was convalescing in the nursing home. Gregory also continued to receive, both directly and indirectly from a variety of staff members, mixed messages about his right to pursue an intimate sexual relationship.

## PROBLEM BEHAVIOR OR A GOD GIVEN RIGHT?

### When Sexuality Is a Problem

Just as it is important to remain open minded about institutionalized older adults' abilities to engage in satisfying sexual behaviors and relationships, it is equally important to stand vigilant and recognize that situations *can* and *do* arise in which such sexual behavior can be inappropriate and potentially damaging to elderly patients (Hodson & Skeen, 1994), and even to staff members and visitors to the institution. The impact of debilitating dementias such as Alzheimer's disease, vascular dementia, and Huntington's Chorea, psychotic disorders such as schizophrenia and bipolar disorder (whose symptoms may become less responsive to medication with age), and entrenched personality disorders can lead to lowered impulse control and the emergence of inappropriate sexual behaviors. It often becomes the job of the clinician, either as staff member or outside consultant, to ascertain the appropriateness of sexual behavior among elderly residents. Even when a behavior is deemed clearly inappropriate, it sometimes becomes more difficult to determine how to manage patients' behavior without imposing undue restrictions on their personal freedom.

Edward

Edward was a 73-year-old white man who has lived in a long-term-care home for the past 10 years. He suffers from vascular dementia, and both his long-term and short-term memory are significantly impaired. Although Edward can ambulate independently, he speaks in sentence fragments and requires assistance for activities of daily living including dressing and personal care. He has been divorced for over 15 years and his three adult children have disowned him. Apparently, Edward had a history of child abuse. He reportedly beat his children repeatedly, and he had been arrested in middle age for exposing himself to a minor. Although it remained unclear what exactly precipitated the breakup of his marriage, staff members assumed that his wife and children grew tired of this inappropriate and predatory behavior. It also remained unclear to what extent Edward engaged in inappropriate sexual behavior—without being caught by the authorities. His records also indicate that he never received, or was required to receive, psychological counseling of any kind.

With the worsening of his dementia, Edward's impulse control was significantly eroded. Various members of the staff experienced or observed Edward's inappropriate behavior while in the nursing home. Despite repeated requests not to do so, Edward would sit in the lounge or in the cafeteria and pull his pants down to his thighs, exposing himself to others. When asked to pull his pants up and cover himself, however, he would summarily comply. After a few months of this behavior, Edward began to lower his pants and make inappropriate comments to staff members. He would ask nursing staff to "touch me" or to "give me blow job." At other times he would look at female staff members and state loudly, "nice tits" or "I want to fuck you." Within a few weeks, his behavior escalated to asking female patients, in addition to female staff members, to touch him or kiss him. Staff were always present when Edward made such inappropriate advances and were able to intercede. It was unclear whether Edward would have taken more active measures to have his requests met if he were unattended.

A critical incident arose during the holiday season when a number of schoolchildren arrived at the nursing home to sing some Christmas carols. When he was escorted into the common room to watch the concert, Edward pointed at one of the schoolgirls and said, "Nice tits. Want some.... Touch me." The alarmed staff member removed Edward from the room within seconds. The girl was talking with other friends at the time and, on questioning, had not heard what had been said to her. The staff called an emergency team meeting immediately to decide how to assess and to manage Edward's behavior. Staff members were frightened for the safety of the patients, and particularly for the safety of young children who might be visiting.

During the team meeting, staff members were shocked to learn that this incident was precipitated by a series of inappropriate events. Although each event was documented in Edward's file, the staff members generally were unaware of the incidents observed by each other, even when they were from the same shift or worked on the same wing. The first order of business in the team meeting was to gather all available information about Edward's inappropriate behavior, and to observe any patterns in its escalation. Edward's move from exposing himself to making direct sexual comments and requests coincided with a ministroke and a further decline in mental status. Significant time was spent discussing the fact that except for exposing himself, Edward never physically forced himself on another patient or staff member. Staff members also reported that although Edward could be redirected for a few minutes, his severely impaired memory prevented him from remembering the reprimand. He could be found to engage in the same problem behavior a few minutes or hours later.

The staff decided that they had to keep lines of communication open to prevent the disclosure of vital information in the future, and to limit Edward's interaction to a wing of the nursing home that housed only male patients. (He had not initiated any inappropriate sexual behavior with men.) Edward also would require one-on-one observation whenever he went to the cafeteria or to group events. However, because of the limitations on staff members' already limited time and resources, Edward would sometimes be forced to eat meals in his own wing or room, and would not be able to attend all scheduled group events. All visitors would be informed to remain within designated areas in order to avoid exposing Edward to other young children or adults.

Staff members also debated about whether they were more disturbed by this patient's behavior because he was a man and not a woman. Many staff members noted that Edward had not physically forced himself on anyone; he had only made verbal comments and requests. The counterpoint was raised that regardless of his sex, these verbal accosts impinged on the personal boundaries of others. Even though staff members were trained to handle such situations, other residents and visitors certainly were not. Because the best predictor of future behavior is past behavior, Edward's prior criminal record, coupled with his current lack of impulse control, did not bode well for his ability to manage inappropriate sexual impulses in the future. Ultimately, the staff had to make a difficult decision between protecting the comfort and safety of other patients and visitors, and maintaining Edward's individual freedom and his ability to ambulate freely about the complex. Because Edward was not capable of making the choice to behave appropriately with women, the staff was forced to make that choice for him.

### Antonia

Antonia was a 66-year-old female patient who suffered from paranoid schizophrenia. She had been in and out of institutions and nursing homes for most of her adult life. Both of her parents had passed away, and her only surviving relative was a niece who visited only irregularly. Antonia's psychotic symptoms also had become more resistant to treatment with psychotropic medications. Her health care providers were becoming anxious that increasing the doses of her medication would result in dangerous side effects and little change in her symptoms. Currently, Antonia believes that her physician is the Devil and that her niece is Jesus incarnate. She is ambulatory and requires only minimal assistance with activities of daily living. Antonia had been attending group therapy and music therapy regularly until she became increasingly paranoid that other patients and staff members wanted to steal her possessions and invade her thoughts.

One staff member noticed that Antonia had begun to spend a lot of her free time on the men's wing of the nursing home. Notably, however, she would not sit and talk with other men on the unit. Instead, she would lurk around corners and appear to spy on some of the men who were more disabled than she. A male patient approached one of the nursing staff and said that Antonia had been "sitting too close" to him and had been asking lots of "strange questions." He refused to elaborate further as to what she had said to him, but indicated that he did not like her to be spending so much time on their floor. Alerted to this potentially inflammatory behavior, the staff member then observed Antonia accosting other men on the unit. On one occasion, she saw Antonia rub her hand briefly against another man's genitals. He appeared shocked and bemused, and she left as quickly as she appeared.

When confronted about this behavior, Antonia denied that anything had happened. She was counseled that touching other residents without their permission was unacceptable behavior, and that if she touched another patient she would lose privileges on the ward. Because medication and supportive psychotherapy were not effective in alleviating many of her symptoms, this behavioral approach (i.e., a token economy) was employed to help manage her acting out. Interestingly, members of the treatment team did not find Antonia's behavior as alarming as the behavior of male patients who engaged in inappropriate sexual behavior. It was as though her sex as a woman made her advances appear more innocuous and even humorous. When treatment team members were asked to consider how alarmed they would be if this behavior were initiated by a male patient toward a female patient, the staff members quickly recognized their gender bias and redoubled their efforts to manage Antonia's sexual acting out.

## Managing Inappropriate Behavior

Managing an institutionalized, elderly patient's inappropriate sexual behavior can be difficult, at best. However, a number of guidelines can be offered to cope with these challenging, if not unusual or atypical, situations. Clinicians can be advised to:

1. Employ a team approach. Gathering information is essential in order to ascertain the appropriateness of the patient's behavior and to generate hypotheses as to its possible origin or escalation.

2. Value all team members' input equally. Ideally, members of the team will include everyone in the institution with whom the patient has direct contact, such as psychologists, nurses, psychiatrists, internists, receptionists, volunteers, nutritionists, social workers, occupational therapists, physical therapists, and administrators.

3. Explore the patient's history regarding sexual behavior. Be alert for any criminal record or evidence of any potential illegal or deviant behaviors.

4. Determine if underlying stressors such as undiagnosed medical problems (e.g., a urinary infection), a perceived loss of independence related to sudden physical decline, the loss of a significant other, or even a room change or change in staffing spurred the occurrence of inappropriate sexual behavior. Sexual acting out often masks elderly residents' responses to pain, fear, instability, and loss of control.

5. Ensure that the patient's sexual behavior is evaluated on the basis of the actual, observed problem behavior and its effect on others, and not on staff members' own fears, insecurities, or religious beliefs. Also make sure that both male and female instigators are evaluated without gender bias. Male patients who engage in inappropriate sexual behaviors often are viewed as sinister and predatory, whereas female patients who engage in similar behaviors are often viewed as hapless and even humorous.

6. Set firm limits with both patients and staff members. If a patient behaves inappropriately, it automatically is unacceptable behavior and sanctions and preventive measures should be enforced. Because some staff members may find one such behavior (e.g., masturbating in a public area) particularly alarming and offensive whereas others may not be as egregiously offended, treatment team members should be counseled to be uniform in their approach to the problem. Personal feelings should not influence the manner in which a problem behavior is dealt with; an objective and effective plan for specific action should already be in place. In other words, all staff members should aim to provide the same standard of care.

7. Inform patients verbally that their actions are inappropriate, even if a patient has a severely limited mental status and cannot understand what is being said. It is beneficial for all staff members involved to concretize and objectify the problem, and it is helpful for other patients who may be witness to the incident. It lets other residents know that appropriate actions have been taken, that their welfare is acknowledged, that patients who may be severely demented are treated fairly and with respect, and that all residents are expected to engage in behaviors within appropriate limits.

8. Consider the safety of other patients and visitors to the facility when making decisions about the management of a patient's problem behavior.

9. Use the least restrictive measures to prevent patients with impaired mental status and poor impulse control from engaging in inappropriate sexual behaviors. For example, it is preferable to allow patients who are

ambulatory to roam freely in a monitored, locked unit instead of drugging them into submission (Fox, 1980) or physically restraining them in a karol chair.

10. Be prepared that staff members who provide primary care are already likely to have significant demands placed on them to monitor a number of patients. These vital staff members should be encouraged to work with administrators and with each other to provide flexible scheduling, multiple break times, and a varied work routine. Staff psychologists often find themselves in a unique position to help foster such mutual cooperation and respect.

11. Monitor staff members' responses to patients who are engaging in sexually inappropriate behavior carefully. Encourage staff members to vent their feelings appropriately in a private forum. Provide emotional and instrumental support, and continuing education as needed.

12. As a mental health professional, maintain your own support system, both inside and outside of the institution. Because a staff therapist is likely to hold multiple roles, it is vital that clinicians make it a priority to monitor and process their own reactions to a number of potentially emotionally charged situations. Ultimately, clinicians must tend to their own needs before they can tend to those of others.

## ASSESSMENT OF RELEVANT ISSUES

### Ethical and Legal Dilemmas

In addition to the difficulties inherent in managing sexual behavior within an institutional setting, clinicians often are asked to make or to mediate decisions that pose decisive moral, ethical, medical, family, religious, and legal dilemmas. Questions often arise about *who* is allowed or entitled to make decisions for an institutionalized elderly person's care. Questions also may arise about whose input is required versus summarily requested, and about which staff members are able to make legally binding decisions about treatment planning.

It may be necessary to turn to administrators or legal counsel to delineate the roles that legal guardians, adult children, physicians, psychiatrists, psychologists, social workers, nurses, and administrators play in making legally binding decisions. Rules also vary from state to state, and among private, public, and Veterans Administration long-term institutions. Legal guardianship, which may be held by the state, family members, or federal agency, may apply to all aspects of patient care to financial matters. Because of confusion about these issues, concerns about malpractice suits, and potential civil suits over inheritances and other monies, legal counsel is often unfortunately a requisite part of patient care. Some lawyers specialize in geriatric care issues, and may already be under employ at an institution as an outside consultant. Be sure, too, to verify the credentials of any lawyer or agency who claims to have expertise in elder issues; in certain situations clinicians may find themselves held legally responsible for decisions based on inaccurate information garnered from a poorly trained legal professional.

Competency and Medical Issues

A common concern that often is shared by both staff members and family members is whether an elderly resident is competent to make clear, rational decisions for her- or himself. Competency itself is a complicated issue that incorporates aspects of psychological, medical, functional, and legal status. In some states, only psychiatrists and medical doctors can make such a determination. In others, psychologists and social workers can make such a ruling. Different professionals also are entitled to make such a determination in public and private settings. In any case, however, mental health practitioners such as psychologists should regard their expertise as unique and vital. Clinicians should draw their own conclusions about a patient's competence, and present both objective and subjective evidence to support their view.

No clear-cut guidelines are offered by any professional psychological organization (e.g., the American Psychological Association) regarding assessment of patient competence. However, a number of geropsychologists (e.g., Ables et al., 1998) have suggested that a variety of measures and an analysis of various clinical observations be used to assist in making such an assessment. These primary assessment tools include:

- Mini-mental state exam (MMSE; Folstein, Folstein, & McHugh, 1975). The MMSE serves as a useful thumbnail sketch of a patient's mental abilities, and provides a familiar, objective measure that is recognized among many professionals from a variety of disciplines.
- Assessment of activities of daily living (e.g., Lawton's Instrumental Activities of Daily Living Scale; Lawton & Brody, 1969). It is helpful to gather information from the patient's significant others as well as staff members to gather an appropriate appraisal of the resident's abilities to care for him- or herself. The use of a team approach, and good relationships with primary care workers, will allow for the most accurate assessment.
- Mattis Dementia Rating Scale (DRS; Mattis, 1973). The DRS is unique in that it allows for an assessment of different aspects of intellectual and cognitive functioning. It also provides an objective overall score that may be recognized readily among other professionals. The caveat with this instrument is that it also is best used only as an overall screening measure, particularly if a patient scores along the "cutoff" point for dementia.
- Other neuropsychological testing where appropriate (e.g., if the DRS score is at approximately the cutoff point for dementia and little is known about the dementia's origin or rate of progression), such as the California Verbal Learning Test (CVLT). The CVLT can be useful in determining dementia etiology, as well as capacities for short- and long-term memory.
- A mental status examination that includes an assessment of the capacity

for self-awareness, ego strength, an awareness of body boundaries, and reality testing. Atypical but helpful questions include, "If you were lost in the [Denver] airport, you only had one dollar in your pocket, and you wanted to come back here, what would you do?"

- A review of medical concerns. It has been noted that underlying medical conditions such as urinary track infections have been responsible for impaired mental status among older adults (Lerner, Hedera, Koss, & Stuckey, 1997). It also is vital to separate the effects of long-term decline in mental status (caused by dementia or chronic mental illness) from the short-term effects of delirium, which often calls for immediate medical intervention.

Sometimes a global pattern of impairment emerges, whereas at other times one specific area of impairment within an otherwise normal-looking picture is enough to raise concerns about patient competence. Additionally, some patients will display severe impairment in certain areas, yet be regarded as fully competent. For example, many patients recovering from strokes or amputations may require almost total care for their activities of daily living (ADLs), but remain completely cognitively intact. Other patients suffering from chronic mental illness such as paranoid schizophrenia may be completely self-sufficient in terms of bathing, grooming, and feeding themselves within the context of the institution, but they may display significantly impaired reality testing and a lack of regard for others' body boundaries and be ruled incompetent.

Sometimes the assessment of competence and the inappropriateness of a sexual behavior is clear. Elderly residents who are deemed incompetent as a result of global changes from advanced dementia have been known to seek out oral sex (e.g., McLean, 1994) or intercourse from multiple, non-consenting, or otherwise unavailable partners, or they may become easy "targets" for more cognitively intact, sexual predators both inside and outside of the institution. In contrast, situations may arise in which patients are declared incompetent because of severe impairment in memory (e.g., they may no longer be able to speak, they do not recognize family members), but they may be permitted to engage in sexual activity primarily because their means of expression takes the form of less invasive activity and because they are granted "approval" from staff and caregivers.

## Emma and Kermit

Emma was an 82-year-old resident of a nursing home. She suffers from advanced Alzheimer's dementia. About 2 months into her stay at the nursing home, she began to hold hands and hug a male patient, Kermit, who lived on her floor and who suffered from the same disorder. Although Emma and Kermit were unable to communicate any longer to anyone, they would shuffle toward each other each morning after breakfast, and sit quietly together in the lobby for a few hours each day. Neither patient attempted to touch other patients or staff members, and other patients did not appear concerned about their physical interactions with each other. In this particular case, staff members and family members decided that no "harm" was being done as both residents were single. The residents' adult children agreed with staff members and felt strongly that this nonverbal communication may be quite beneficial and reassuring (e.g., Walz & Blum, 1987) to their otherwise isolated and mute parents.

Familial Concerns

Adult children of institutionalized, elderly patients often become intimately involved in their parents' care. Yet, few of these children have ever had to consider their parents' sexuality at any other time in their lives. Once the traditional oedipal conflict has been resolved, most children necessarily view their parents as asexual beings. While serving as legal guardian, situations sometimes arise in which adult children are asked to make difficult decisions about their impaired elderly parent's room assignments, to "give permission" for their parent to engage in romantic relationships with other patients, or to give their opinions as to whether their parent is competent to make his or her own decisions or not. Horribly complicated issues may emerge in which an elderly parent, who is severely demented, seeks out hugging and kissing with another patient who is moderately cognitively impaired. Although the interaction at first appears to staff members as mutual and beneficial for both parties, they learn quickly that the elderly parent who initiated the relationship is married, with a physically disabled spouse who lives in a rehabilitation center in a neighboring state. Many adult children of such residents do the very best they can to manage such difficult emotional issues. Many take advantage of help from peers and professionals to make sometimes more lenient and sometimes more restrictive decisions in the best interest of their elderly parent.

Other adult children can be observed to become overly involved and controlling in their parent's life in the institution, while others opt to remove themselves completely from any decision making and deprive staff members from their typically insightful input. Some common issues can cloud the judgment of adult children regarding the sexual activity of their parents in a nursing home facility. These may include:

- Fear that their parent will be taken advantage of emotionally by a new partner. Many adult children project their own fears of loss for their aging parent (through death or decline in mental state) onto the situation, and reason that their elderly parent will not be able to withstand the loss of a potential suitor in the immediate future.
- Strong religious views that may or may not be consistent with those of their parent regarding sexual activities. Religious beliefs may be particularly strong regarding sexuality outside of marriage and masturbation. While the religious beliefs held by the resident's children *must* be re-

spected, it often is helpful to help these adult children base decisions for their elderly parent on their understanding of, and respect for, their *parent's* religious beliefs.

- Financial concerns that if their elderly parent becomes involved with and subsequently marries a visitor or resident, they may lose some or all of their inheritance. Adult children also may fear that if their elderly parent is cognitively impaired, he or she may be taken advantage of financially by more cognitively intact suitors.
- Unresolved issues regarding the death of a parent. If the elderly parent in the nursing home is a widow, the adult child may cling to the belief that the surviving parent should not seek out another relationship out of respect for the marriage vows to the deceased spouse. This is commonly observed when the adult child has not fully mourned the death of the parent or when he or she somehow blames the widowed parent for the other parent's death.
- Personality disorders or deep-seated conflicts in which the adult children may have difficulty establishing their own romantic relationship or may have dissatisfaction in their current romantic relationship. Because of conscious or unconscious feelings of competition and sadism, the adult children do not want their elderly parent to "be happy" when they themselves are not.

Managing the conflicts that such adult children bring to the treatment setting can sometimes be as difficult as managing the practical issues involved in their own parent's sexual activities. Adult children often respond well when they are encouraged to participate in long-term planning and to discuss their thoughts and concerns with treatment team members and with other adult children of elderly residents. Thanking these often reluctant caregivers for their time and participation can allay many of their anxieties and allow these children to focus more clearly on the issues at hand. At times it is necessary for staff members to enforce limits, and ensure that the adult children recognize that while their views are to be respected, they may or may not be different from the views of the trained professionals who care for their parent on a daily basis. Knowing that they can rely on a professional to help them make choices also can help minimize feelings of guilt or confusion among emotionally distraught adult caregivers.

## Practical Issues

Many authors maintain that nursing homes are devoid of opportunities for sexual expression (Fox, 1980). Effective comparisons have been made between prisons and their allowances for conjugal visits, and nursing homes and their outright lack of allowances for such visits (Hodson & Skeen, 1994). Most believe that these restrictive environments primarily reflect the negative attitudes held by staff members and the oppressive administrative policies enacted simply to make things "easier" for staff members (Hobson, 1984; McCartney, Izeman, Rogers, & Cohen, 1987). Others suggest that these problems could be ameliorated simply by instituting privacy rooms (Monks, 1975; Wallace, 1992) or minimizing the frequency of nightly bed checks (Wasow & Loeb, 1978). Comments also have been made that traditional hospital beds are simply too narrow to permit two people to comfortably engage in sexual activity (Wasow & Loeb, 1978). Thus, in an ideal setting, institutions would engender more permissive administrative policies that do not label any sexual behaviors as "problem behaviors," provide double beds for all residents, offer a privacy room for residents to engage in masturbation or intercourse, provide less frequent bed checks for patients who seek privacy in the evenings, and foster interaction between male and female patients. However, it appears that as much as some administrators may be guilty of enacting restrictive policies to simplify their duties and concerns, many gerontologists wish to provide an equally "simple" solution to a very complicated problem.

A number of practical issues detract significantly from the utility of the aforementioned suggestions. Because the need for bed space is increasing rapidly in nursing home settings, many institutions are not equipped to provide double beds for its residents, much less single, private rooms. Many nursing homes offer a combination of accommodations ranging from single rooms, double rooms, to rooms housing four patients. Some administrators provide single rooms to patients who require the most acute care, others provide single rooms to the patients who can afford to pay the associated higher price, and others provide single rooms based on availability and patient request. Certainly no national standards or guidelines are set regarding such decisions or policies. Other patients are advised to sleep in the proverbial, narrow hospital bed because they need support from bed rails or from the ability of the bed to incline.

The use of a privacy room poses other challenges for nursing home staff members. One limitation is that of space; one private room must be equipped with a double bed and a locked door. This also represents a space that cannot be used to store supplies, function as a recreation area for all patients, or to serve as living quarters for patients. Although some administrators are opposed to the idea simply on its principle, others fear for the loss of revenue, whereas others fear that the legal liabilities related to the use of the privacy room are simply too great. Some have posed questions such as, "Who would decide who was capable of using the privacy room? How will mutual consent be determined? How long could a person or a couple use the room? What kind of safety risks are posed if the residents are behind a locked door and there is some kind of medical or psychiatric emergency?" More pointedly, many primary care nurses ask, "What if they need help taking their clothes on and off? What if they fall out of bed? Who will be left to clean up after a patient masturbates or has intercourse?—We will." When asked about less frequent bed checks, both administrators and nurses balk for reasons of health and safety. In sum, the ideas proposed are theoretically sound, but are very difficult to put into practice for a variety of practical, as well as some prejudicial, reasons. There appear to be no simple answers.

## MODEL PROGRAMS AND CURRENT POLICIES

Although many institutions do not appear to be moving toward more permissive policies toward elderly sexuality, a number of nursing homes do promote an open discussion of sexuality among its residents, staff members, and family members of their residents. Family members and older adults themselves also can select long-term care based on certain criteria that allow for greater freedom of sexual expression. Some questions that one might consider when selecting a nursing home include:

- Are men and women relegated to discrete aspects (i.e., wings or floors) of the facility? What opportunities are there for social interaction between men and women (e.g., dances, dining, concerts, bingo, crafts, exercise)?
- Can husbands and wives share a room? Will they have two double beds or could arrangements be made to share a double bed? What happens if one spouse becomes ill and requires more intensive care?
- Is a privacy room available for residents' use? Is it available for masturbation, intercourse, and even for dates or card games? Do residents have to sign up in advance? Is medical assistance available? Is there a lock on the door, and if so, what requirements are needed to use it?
- Do staff members receive education and training on how to interpret and discuss issues related to elderly sexuality?
- Is there a written policy for the institution regarding sexual activity and expression?
- Do residents have opportunities to openly and objectively discuss sexual issues such as dating (Hodson & Skeen, 1994)? Can they receive education about possible changes in sexual physiology with aging and about HIV prevention (Kendig & Adler, 1990)?
- Are opportunities available to increase self-esteem and experience sensual pleasures through frequent visits from hairdressers, barbers, clothing consultants (Malatesta, Chambless, Pollack, & Cantor, 1988), and massage therapists?
- Can residents bring their own furniture including beds and bed linens to increase a sense of home, familiarity, and sensuality?

## SUMMARY

As noted, issues regarding elderly sexuality within an institutional setting are multifaceted. Different challenges are posed to elderly residents, their adult children, administrators, and nursing home staff members including mental health practitioners. Many clinicians initially fear working within an institutional setting, but often find their work challenging but rewarding. Issues of elderly sexuality may come as a surprise, and psychologists often find themselves in the role of educator, arbitrator, legal advisor, support group leader, and case manager. Psychologists working within nursing homes often find that they provide as much education to staff members about elderly sexuality as they do actually working therapeutically with elderly residents in this area themselves. Issues of competence, prejudice, and medical, legal, religious, familial, and practical concerns must all be addressed in order to make appropriate recommendations. Because nursing homes are believed to be among the institutions most devoid of human contact and sensuality (Fox, 1980; Hodson & Skeen, 1994; Walz & Blum, 1987), psychologists also are in a unique position to foster appropriate sensual and sexual expression in an otherwise sterile environment.

# 5

# The Impact of Disability
# and Chronic Illness

*Older adults both inside and outside of nursing homes cope with chronic illnesses. More than one in three community-living older adults report that a chronic illness poses some limitation in their otherwise normal activities (Dorgan, 1995).*

## SEXUALITY WITHIN THE CONTEXT OF DISABILITIES

Disability can be thought of loosely as any medical or psychological condition that impairs a person's normal range of functioning. Disabilities can be acute, such as a myocardial infarction that presents as a one-time incident (that may or may not lead to a complete recovery), or they can be chronic, as in the case of rheumatoid arthritis occurring as a lifelong illness. Both acute and chronic illnesses wage an assault on an elderly person's physical, cognitive, and psychological sense of self. Elderly adults are often faced with the challenge of adapting to life with one or more chronic illnesses or adapting to life as a caregiver of a partner coping with such an illness. The emotional toll sometimes can be so great that patients, caregivers, and health care providers themselves neglect to acknowledge the impact of these illnesses on an older adult's sex life. Societal stereotypes that sexuality is reserved for the young and the healthy provide additional barriers to successful adaptation to these life challenges.

### Successful Coping

In order to cope successfully with any disability, an elderly adult must:

1. Acknowledge the presence of the disability or illness
2. Mourn the loss of any physical, cognitive, or emotional abilities
3. Have a realistic appraisal of the illness via informed health care providers and become an active participant in a treatment plan designed to alleviate symptoms and maximize independence

4. Recognize that sexuality can continue to be an important part of life, regardless of whether he or she is disabled or is coping with a chronic illness

An individual must first acknowledge the presence of a disorder in order to cope effectively. Denial is a primitive defense that will allow an older adult to believe that things are operating on the status quo, but it requires a great expense of energy and is not effective in the long run. Some degree of ego strength is required for an elderly adult to acknowledge that his or her physical or psychic sense of self has been violated or changed. Also, the very nature of certain chronic illnesses, such as Alzheimer's disease and schizophrenia, can limit the elderly person's ability to recognize the presence of an illness. In these situations, the caregiver is often faced with the task of identifying the presence of a disorder and seeking help for his or her elderly spouse, relative, or partner.

Once elderly patients recognize that they are faced with some life changes, they are better equipped to mourn any losses and reestablish a sense of self based on their internal versus external attributes. A trusting therapeutic relationship can ease the pain of admission and allow for the articulation and venting of emotions in response to the presence of a sometimes crippling disease. Life review, psychodynamic, and cognitive–behavioral therapies can all be useful in allowing elderly patients to experience anger, sadness, helplessness, curiosity, rage, and resignation in the mourning process. Both elderly patients and their mental health care practitioners should recognize that even though many older adults do suffer from chronic illness, advanced age itself is not an automatic "death sentence" from activities of daily living or satisfaction in sexual activities.

The Importance of Patient Education

Even though mourning can be considered a psychological process, the presence of accurate information about a disorder, including specific medical information about its etiology and treatment, is essential in order for an elderly person to adapt most effectively. Providing information about the course of an illness can concretize an otherwise ambiguous life event, and provide necessary structure and expectations for patient progress. Many older adults are not well informed about the nature of their illnesses, much less the impact of their disorders on their sexual functioning. Empirical studies suggest that the vast majority of patients fail to receive any information about sexuality in relation to their acute or chronic illness (e.g., Walker, Osgood, Richardson, & Ephross, 1998).

Even though geropsychologists are not medical personnel, they have the responsibility to be familiar with the diseases that their patients may be dealing with, and to be available to discuss the impact of these diseases on sexual functioning. In the words of one prominent geropsychologist, "we must wear many professional 'hats' in order to best serve the needs of our patients." In the following sections, a number of common ailments experienced in late life are presented. Certain medical aspects of these disorders are highlighted in order to provide the appropriate background for mental health care practitioners.

## ARTHRITIS

Estimates suggest that up to 48% of older adults suffer from arthritis, including rheumatoid and osteoarthritis (Dorgan, 1995). Writing, walking, and other activities of daily living becoming increasingly difficult and painful. Patients may feel ashamed of the appearance of their hands, which may become misshapen over the course of the disease. A vicious cycle often ensues in which an elderly patient experiences pain when walking or moving an extremity, which leads to a general lack of physical activity, to muscle stiffness and reduced joint lubrication, to even more pain in response to movement. In sum, elderly adults with arthritis often limit their activities of daily living, including participation in sexual activity.

For an elderly person with arthritis, sexual relations can become more painful than enjoyable. Many patients describe experiencing the most pain and stiffness during the evening, the night, and the early morning, i.e., the times most people reserve for love making (Badeau, 1995). Difficulties in flexion of the hips, knees, and back can cause significant pain during intercourse and require older adults to seek out new, and potentially unfamiliar and threatening, sexual positions. Even if an elderly patient cannot engage in intercourse, satisfying him or her with manual stimulation may be difficult because of pain and general lack of mobility in the hands and fingers.

To complicate the issue further, the medications often prescribed to reduce the pain and swelling associated with arthritis may reduce interest in sex. The steroids prescribed to control swelling often provoke impotence in male patients. Other side effects from such medications include hair loss, hair growth in undesirable places, and weight gain. It often is difficult to feel attractive and desirable when one is in pain, impotent, and believes that he or she is physically unattractive. Unfortunately, a pervasive exists in the medical community suggests that arthritis is a common chronic illness that does not affect an older adult's sexual functioning (e.g., Golan & Chong, 1992; Kellett, 1991).

Some suggestions can be made for elderly patients with arthritis who would like to engage in satisfying sexual relations. Sexual activity can be pursued during the daytime hours (when pain generally is less intense), and older adults often feel relieved when they give themselves "permission" to unplug the phone and ignore the doorbell for a few hours. Warm baths to loosen muscles and to foster intimacy and pleasure in itself can be incorporated as foreplay. Alternative positions for vaginal intercourse can have the woman lie on her side with her knees drawn up. Some researchers even suggest that sexual activity can stimulate the natural production of endorphins and corticosteroids. These neurochemicals are natural pain relievers whose effect may last for hours after the conclusion of sexual activity (Badeau, 1995). Sexual activity also may result in a more relaxed musculoskeletal system (Butler, Lewis, Hoffman, & White-head, 1994) and presumably a lesser experience of pain.

From a psychological perspective, elderly patients coping with arthritis also must feel free to refrain from sexual activity if it is too painful or uncomfortable. When told about their options for sexual activity, some elderly patients may feel guilty or like "a quitter" if they do not engage actively in vaginal intercourse with their partner. It is vital that patients with arthritis, like any chronic illness or disability, engage in sexual behavior that is comfortable for them, and not feel pressured to engage in sex to meet the expectations of a physician or therapist. Couples therapy also can improve communication between partners and establish new and enjoyable patterns of sexual relations that may incorporate sensual as well as sexual activities.

## DEPRESSION

### Differential Symptoms among Older Adults

Depression is one of the more common ailments among older adults. Approximately 1% of elderly adults are estimated to suffer from major depression, and nearly 20% of elderly adults in the community report depressive symptoms that meet the criteria for dysthymic disorder or adjustment disorder with depressive features (Ables et al., 1998). Even though a landmark meta-analysis revealed that psychological and pharmacological treatments for depression are just as effective among older, as compared to younger, adults (Scogin & McElreath, 1994), the differential symptom presentation of depression among older adults may make the initial diagnosis somewhat difficult. Specifically, older adults may manifest depression via somatic complaints versus general complaints about feeling sad, depressed, or "blue." Older adults, as compared to younger adults, also are more prone to display cognitive impairments and delusions when depressed. (In any responsible discussion of depression among elderly adults, it must be noted that older adults are at greater risk for completed suicide than their younger counterparts, and that suicidal ideation must be explored thoroughly with any elderly patient.) Depression among this cohort also can be caused by a variety of organic problems including medical disorders such as Parkinson's disease or even a urinary track infection. In making an appropriate diagnosis, it is just as important to ask older patients about changes in their sexual habits and interests as it is their younger counterparts. It often is difficult to ascertain whether sexual difficulties among depressed older adults represent a symptom of the depression itself or whether they stem from other medical or psychological problems.

### Issues in Treatment

Clinicians themselves are beginning to display age-appropriate, realistic attitudes toward older adults and their chances for success in response to appropriate treatment (e.g., Hillman et al., 1997). However, sometimes patients and their spouses may have unrealistic expectations for treatment. One patient's wife told her therapist, "Well, if I sleep with him more often ... that should cheer him up and get him out of his funk!" Thus, including the partner in therapy and treatment planning, with appropriate permission from the patient, of course, may be vital. With this arrangement, both parties are encouraged to discuss current changes in their sex life, possible guilt about the etiology of the disorder, and realistic expectations for treatment.

Another aspect of treatment that can impact greatly on a depressed elderly patient's sexual expression is the multitude of side effects that accompany most antidepressant medications. The antidepressant drugs listed in Table 3 have been shown to cause problems with the normal sexual response cycle, including diminished overall arousal and inability to orgasm among both men and women (see Schiavi & Segraves, 1995, for a review).

Popular serotonin reuptake inhibitors (e.g., fluoxetine, sertraline, and paroxetine), which are used widely among depressed older adults because of their low incidence of anticholinergic effects, are responsible for many of these sexual side effects (Butler et al., 1994). The pervasiveness of these debilitating side effects has been documented extensively. Findings from double-blind studies suggest that up to 90% of men taking 50 mg or more of clomipramine (Monteiro et al., 1987), and up to 75% of men taking fluoxetine (Walker et al., 1993) were unable to experience orgasm. The use of alternative medications such as bupropion or Wellbutrin, or a decrease in dosage of the current medication, may help alleviate patients' sexual dysfunction (Butler et al., 1994). In sum, psychotherapists should be well aware of any medications that their patients are taking for depression, and both ask and inform their patients about any possible side effects. There *are* ways to combat medications' side effects.

Other antidepressant medications, including selective serotonin reuptake inhibitors such as Prozac, may induce the opposite effect intended in its use among elderly patients. One such side effect is that of manic behavior. Although this manic response is generally rare, it may present itself in unusual ways and may reveal underlying sexual frustrations or conflicts.

## Mario

Mario was a 68-year-old man diagnosed with severe depression. He took a daily dose of Prozac in conjunction with his weekly psychotherapy. After a few

TABLE 3. Antidepressant Medications
that Can Interfere with Sexual Functioning

| Drug name | Brand or trade name | Drug name | Brand or trade name |
|-----------|---------------------|-----------|---------------------|
| Fluoxetine | Prozac | Imipramine | Tofranil |
| Sertraline | Zoloft | Phenelzine | Nardil |
| Paroxetine | Paxil | Clomipramine | Anafranil |

months of treatment, Mario became manic as a side effect of his medication. His speech became rapid and pressured, he became visibly agitated, he became grandiose, and his judgment became impaired. During a therapy session, he showed his psychologist a note written by his wife. Mario said that he promised his wife he would tell "his story," even though he believed it was just nothing. Apparently, Mario had begun to cross the street haphazardly, barely avoiding being hit by passing cars. When asked if his wife and his therapist had reason to be concerned about him getting hurt in traffic, he responded, "Well, I just dare them to hit me.... I feel like they would just bounce off of me ... look at me, I'm a strong guy for my age! See those muscles!"

Mario also said that his wife got very upset with him because he had begun to flirt with waitresses when they went out to dinner. "You know, I'm not hurting anybody. I'm just having fun!" His therapist calmly asked about the incident in detail, and asked Mario why he thought his wife got so upset when he did not stop; he admitted that the restaurant owner had come to their table to ask him to "keep it down" and "to keep his hands to himself." Mario also admitted that he had gotten up a few times during dinner to "make a speech" to celebrate the occasion. On consultation with his psychiatrist and input from Mario, his medication was adjusted.

Once his dosage had been adjusted and he was no longer manic, Mario recognized easily that he should not have touched the waitress without her permission. He also admitted that he wished he could continue to feel so "high" instead of feeling depressed. He also had enough ego strength to recognize that his desire to be desirable to women represented an underlying conflict in his own marriage, and his difficulties in feeling "old, weak, and unmanly." With the help of his therapist, Mario was able to work on these issues underlying his depression, and develop more positive coping strategies.

## DIABETES

Diabetes is a chronic illness that affects nearly 1 in 10 elderly men and women (Dorgan, 1995). Although most people who experience adult-onset diabetes can control its course with diet, medication, and exercise, diabetes often requires strict adherence to a treatment regimen. Diabetes also can result in significant anxiety and misunderstanding among its sufferers because it is commonly linked to sexual dysfunction in both men and women. Specifically, diabetes has been recognized as the number one organic cause of male impotence (Deacon, Minichiello, & Plummer, 1995), and its effects are most pronounced among elderly men (Badeau, 1995). Impotence arises from vascular and neurological changes. It is important to note that for these men who suffer from diabetes related impotence, underlying sexual urges, interest, and opportunities for sensual pleasure are not diminished in any physiological way.

The impact of diabetes on female sexuality has typically been ignored, both clinically and in research trials (Badeau, 1995). Myths persist in the medical community that diabetes has little impact on female sexuality (e.g., Golan & Chong, 1992; Kellett, 1991). Among women, sexual dysfunction can result from a lack of blood flow to the clitoris and vagina during sexual arousal. Atrophy of the uterus and ovaries also has been observed (Golan & Chong, 1992). Although women may continue to experience orgasm, an overall decrease in frequency of orgasm and an increase in the amount of manual stimulation required to achieve orgasm result from diabetes. These changes in sexual response are real, and should not be ignored or overlooked by physical or mental health care providers.

### Amputations as Complications

Another aspect of diabetes that is often not discussed in relation to elderly sexuality is that of limb amputation. Diabetes often causes vascular difficulties, and typically lower extremities such as toes, feet, and even lower legs must be amputated as a result of poor blood flow, infection, or gangrene. Amputees overall tend to be elderly; more than 85% of all amputations occur among patients over the age of 60 (Schulz, Williamson, & Bridges, 1991). Coupled with generally ageist attitudes that only young, healthy individuals are entitled to engage in sexual relations, health care providers themselves appear reluctant to discuss changes in sexual attitudes or functioning in response to the loss of a limb (Mulligan & Moss, 1991). Less than 10% of lower extremity amputees reported having any physician-initiated discussion of sexuality after their surgery (Williamson & Walters, 1996).

Regarding sexual activity among amputees, being older and being single were predictive of less participation and satisfaction in sexual relations (Williamson & Walters, 1996). Barriers to sexuality include pain at the site of amputation, embarrassment about not being normal or "whole," and concerns that their partner finds them "defective" or unattractive. Concerns about loss of body integrity are often overlooked among older adult patients, with some members of society and the health care community maintaining the belief that older people should simply expect to experience disability and deformity. Depression also is a common response to amputation, which can impact negatively on sexual functioning. Thus, it appears essential that mental health practitioners provide a source of information and support for elderly amputees who wish to return to their normal sex lives.

### HEART DISEASE

As clinicians and scientists, we recognize that the brain is the seat of our emotions and consciousness, and that it alone oversees the activity and coordination of all organ systems. However, popular culture dictates that our heart is the most important part of our anatomy, which has become imbued with unique spiritual and emotional characteristics. We speak from the bottom of our hearts, follow our hearts, and experience heartache and heartbreak. This muscular organ, only about the size of our fist, has come to represent love, caring, fidelity, courage, and security. We seek out people who are kind hearted and lion hearted. It should come as no surprise that heart disease, experienced by nearly one-third of older adults (Dorgan, 1995), can be interpreted as a central assault to the self. If damage to the heart occurs, patients often wonder if they are still "the same person," with the same beliefs, thoughts, and potential for love. The implications for elderly sexuality in relation to heart disease should not be underestimated from either a medical or psychological standpoint.

Recovering from a Heart Attack

Myocardial infarctions can range from mild incidents that are experienced as being slightly out of breath to severe incidents that lead to severe crushing pains and emergency hospitalizations. In either case, the heart muscle becomes deprived of oxygen and suffers from damage. Once stabilized, patients are allowed to return home to resume normal activities after a course of rehabilitation. For most patients, returning to normal life includes a desire to resume a normal sex life.

Despite excellent medical care and completion of physical rehabilitation programs, fear of another heart attack and performance anxiety can inhibit a heart patient's full return to, and enjoyment in, sexual activity. Other patients respond with anger and frustration when they believe they are no longer able to perform sexually (Papadopoulos, Beaumont, Shelley, & Larrimore, 1983). Anxiety disorders and depression also may develop after a heart attack. For elderly patients, these concerns may be heightened by fears of death and by submission to stereotypical beliefs that older adults, particularly those with "bad tickers," have no need for, or interest in, sexual activity. Empirical research studies confirm that it is the patient's psychological response to the myocardial infarction, and not the severity of the heart attack itself, that is the better predictor of sexual disability (Thompson, 1990).

Providing education about the energy expenditures required for sexual activity and the warning symptoms to be on the alert for during intercourse can be vital in allowing elderly patients to begin to feel comfortable with themselves again. Although a wealth of information is available, medical personnel may not share this information with their patients unless they ask for it directly (Albarran & Bridger, 1997). Elderly patients, adhering to their cohort's general prohibition against discussing sexual issues openly, are apt to be less likely than their younger counterparts to approach their health care providers with questions about resuming sexual relations. Some *general* facts and guidelines regarding sexual activity after a heart attack include (e.g., Albarran & Bridger, 1997; Briggs, 1994; Seidl et al., 1991):

- The energy required to perform sexual intercourse is roughly equivalent to that of briskly climbing two flights of stairs or walking on a treadmill at 3 to 4 miles an hour.

- Recognition that the majority of hypertensive drugs can cause side effects that limit sexual function.
- The use of a couple's "usual" positions during sex is advisable in the early stages of recovery. Changing to novel positions have been shown to increase blood pressure and heart rate. Having the woman "on top" or lying side to side have not been shown to decrease cardiac workload (Hellerstein & Friedman, 1970).
- Having sexual relations with a familiar partner in familiar surroundings with a comfortable room temperature is a consideration. Unusual extremes in heat or cold (from either a hot or cold shower) also can increase cardiac workload.
- Masturbation requires less energy output than sexual intercourse, and can provide stress reduction and sexual fulfillment, particularly in the early stages of recovery.
- Having sex in the morning is desirable because of the benefits of a full night of sleep.
- Taking prescription medications such as nitroglycerin before sex may prevent chest pain.
- Waiting to engage in sex 3 hours after eating or drinking is vital. Blood vessels dilate in order to digest food and in response to alcohol.
- Recovering patients should expect some discomfort during intercourse including shortness of breath, sweating, and fatigue.
- Knowing the "warning signs" for stopping sexual activity and consulting a physician is critical. Some of these more serious symptoms include chest pain, heart palpitations, or shortness of breath during intercourse. A failure to return to resting heart rate 7 to 10 minutes after orgasm also is cause for concern.
- The use of foreplay is essential for both physical and emotional preparation for intercourse.
- Consider resuming sexual relations with an emphasis placed on mutual pleasure, without the specific goal of orgasm. Sensate exercises can be particularly helpful in alleviating performance anxiety.

Although mental health practitioners certainly cannot and *should not* attempt to provide advice and direction regarding their patient's physical care, a knowledge base of symptoms and treatment planning is essential. Clinicians often help elderly patients communicate more effectively with their primary health care providers to gain the knowledge and support that they need. Therapists often find themselves freed up to help elderly patients differentiate between realistic concerns and nihilistic fantasies regarding their heart attack and recovery. Partners also can be included in such therapeutic discussions in order to allay their fears and anxieties. Many partners of older adults with heart attacks begin to fear that they are unattractive when their partners hesitate to resume sexual relations. Others have unrealistic expectations about the rate of recovery, the role of medications, or only a limited understanding of their partner's fears and anxieties.

Stroke

Cardiovascular accidents (CVAs) or strokes are another outcropping of heart disease. In this case, a decrease in blood flow to parts of the brain causes tissue damage and transient or permanent changes in functioning. The aftermath of a stroke not only includes physical changes (most commonly paralysis) but also psychological adjustment. In addition to coping with a major medical emergency and potentially drastic changes in physical status, the injury to the brain itself may induce depression, impaired memory, and other changes in mental status. Clinicians must be alert to the synergistic affects of trauma and neuropsychological injury itself. Brain injury resulting from the stroke itself can lead to a loss of interest in sex, although this phenomenon has been observed typically as short lived (Kellett, 1991).

Stroke survivors who lose the ability to speak (i.e., aphasia) may find it particularly difficult to communicate with their partners, much less resume sexual activities. Compounding the problem, many partners and some health care providers do not recognize that the areas governing the production of speech are different than those responsible for the comprehension of speech. A stroke patient who cannot talk does not necessarily lose the ability to understand what is going on around her, or to understand what is being said to her. Talking "down to" or babying a stroke patient with aphasia may further erode the patient's self-esteem and later interest in resuming normal sexual relations. If a patient has become paralyzed, typically occurring on one side of the body (i.e., hemiparesis), suggestions can be made to allow the partially paralyzed partner to participate more fully in sexual activity. Patients may be instructed to lie on pillows on their nonfunctional side, allowing for a greater range of motion with their free hand and leg to caress and hold their partner. Elderly patients also are often comforted to know that no association has been found between sexual activity and the occurrence of subsequent CVAs (Badeau, 1995).

High Blood Pressure

Hypertension is a common chronic illness among older adults; more than 37% of adults over the age of 65 cope with elevated blood pressure (Dorgan, 1995). If untreated, symptoms can include headaches, irritability, fatigue, depression, anxiety, and dizziness. If left untreated, high blood pressure also can lead to CVAs and heart attacks. Although most cases of hypertension can be managed effectively with lifestyle changes and medication, the majority of drugs used to treat high blood pressure have side effects that negatively affect patients' sexual functioning. Many of these drugs also are used for patients recovering from myocardial infarctions and stroke. A listing of some of the more commonly prescribed drugs that have induced sexual dysfunction is given in Table 4 (see also Seidl et al., 1991). It is important to note that these side effects may affect both men and women. Whereas older men commonly experience a loss of interest in sex, difficulties in reaching orgasm, and impotence, older

TABLE 4.  Antihypertensive Medications
that Can Interfere with Sexual Functioning

| Drug | Trade name | Drug | Trade name |
|---|---|---|---|
| Hydrochlorothiazide | HydroDIURIL, Lopressor | Clonidine | Catapres |
| Reserpine | Diupres, Hydropres, Diutensen | Guanethidine | Esimil, Ismelin |
| Chlorothiazide | Aldoclor, Diuril | Prazosin | Minipress |
| Digoxin | Lanoxin, Digibind | Labetalol | Normodyne |
| Spironolactone | Aldactone | Propranolol | Inderal, Inderide |

women are more likely to experience vaginal dryness and a lack of sexual interest. Many health care providers have been accused of being uninformed about these potentially devastating side effects (Briggs, 1994). As noted, it is vital for clinicians to be aware of all medications that their patients are taking.

## INCONTINENCE

Up to one-half of all elderly residents in nursing homes are incontinent (Diokno, Brock, Brown, & Herzog, 1986; McCormack, Newman, Colling, & Pearson, 1992), and more than one-half of all stroke patients have been reported to be incontinent while hospitalized immediately after their CVA (Wade & Hewer, 1985). What may be more surprising is that estimates suggest that up to one-third of all *community-living* older adults in the United States will suffer from urinary incontinence at some point in their lives (Diokno et al., 1986; McCormack, 1992). Although incontinence is one of the most common disorders among older adults, it is one of the least discussed and understood by older adults themselves. Many elderly individuals who are otherwise healthy and active become depressed, anxious, and socially isolated because they do not want to go out in public out of fears of "wetting" or "giving themselves away" by some odor. One can consider the corollary—that incontinence puts significant strain on an elderly person's sense of sexuality and exacerbates any existing concerns about intimacy.

Many older adults assume that incontinence is simply a by-product of aging, and that there is no treatment for this problem. To the contrary, estimates suggest that up to 60% of community-living older adults who experience incontinence can show a complete cessation of, or at least a significant improvement in, their symptoms (Gardner & Fonda, 1994). To assist an older adult in treating incontinence, it becomes important to gain the appropriate medical consultation to identify the specific type of incontinence. Four primary types of loss of bladder and bowel control are: stress incontinence (loss of urine from sneezing, coughing, or lifting in response to pelvic muscle weakness), urge incontinence (preceded by a sudden overwhelming urge to urinate, the patient cannot get to the commode in time), overflow incontinence (in which urine leaks from a distended and overflowing bladder), and reflex incontinence (loss of bladder or bowel control related to a neurological disorder such as Parkinson's disease).

Although influenced by psychological and environmental factors, incontinence typically has its basis in underlying medical problems. Such medical problems are as diverse as stroke, diabetes, obesity, alcohol abuse, pneumonia, prostate gland enlargement, urinary tract infections (UTIs), Alzheimer's disease, Parkinson's disease, and multiple sclerosis. Sometimes conditions in the environment play a role in incontinence, particularly in institutional settings. Some of these situational barriers to bladder and bowel control include toilets without appropriate height supports or hand holds, poor lighting in bathrooms, binding clothing that is difficult to remove quickly, and cold room temperatures. Other older adults may drink multiple cups of caffeinated coffee during a busy morning, or drink too many martinis at one sitting and overflow their bladders inadvertently.

A variety of drugs commonly prescribed to older adults also can induce changes in bowel and bladder habits. Because constipation can lead to bowel obstruction and loss of bowel control, a variety of medications can lead to difficulties with both urinary and fecal incontinence. See Table 5 for a brief review of these drugs and their potential side effects.

From an interpersonal perspective, in addition to causing discomfort and anxiety about circulating freely in public, many older adults with poor bladder or bowel control panic at the thought of being in bed or close to a partner and losing control. Sometimes simply being sure to empty one's bladder before intimate dinners, walks, or interludes is enough to prevent an accident. Elderly male patients are often relieved to learn that it is anatomically impossible for urine to "come out at the same time" as ejaculate when they are with a partner. Other elderly patients experience incontinence on a more global level. They feel infantilized when they have "accidents," "wet" themselves, or need to wear "diapers," and literally accept that this disorder represents a return to a help-

TABLE 5.   Medications that Can Induce
Changes in Bladder and Bowel Habits[a]

| Drug type | Possible side effects |
| --- | --- |
| Antidepressants | Constipation |
| Tranquilizers | Constipation |
| Anticholinergics | Urinary retention, constipation |
| Narcotic pain relievers | Constipation, confusion |
| Diuretics | Frequency and urgency in urination |
| Alpha-adrenergic blockers | Bladder neck relaxation |
| Caffeine | Frequency and urgency in urination |
| Antihypertensives | Unsteady posture |
| Analgesics | Constipation |
| Alcohol | Frequency and urgency in urination |
|  | Unsteady posture |

[a]Adapted from Gardner and Fonda (1994) with permission.

less, sexless stage of life that resembles infancy. It is important for elderly patients to understand that having symptoms of incontinence in no way returns them to an infantile, regressive state; they are simply older adults coping with a medical problem. Education about the disorder, coupled with the ability to discuss overall fears of losing control and independence in a trusting therapeutic relationship, often allows older adults with incontinence to regain their sense of vitality and agency.

For elderly patients who wish to manage their incontinence with conservative measures, aside from medication or surgery, a number of options are available. These behavioral measures may include (e.g., Gardner & Fonda, 1994):

- Kegel exercises for men and women. There are some suggestions that elderly women who engage in regular sexual activity perform natural Kegel exercises that reduce urinary incontinence (Butler et al., 1994).
- Maintaining fluid intake between six and eight glasses of fluid a day, avoiding the use of caffeinated and alcoholic beverages.
- Undergoing behavior training that includes relaxation exercises when in the midst of an urge to urinate, and biofeedback techniques that help promote pelvic muscle control.
- Maintaining a normal body weight to avoid putting additional strain on bladder and bowel muscles.
- Scheduling bathroom times to avoid rushing and to make sure that the bladder and bowel can be completely emptied. Planning a specific time to have a bowel movement in one's morning routine, for example, can lead to increased regularity in bowel habits and thus decrease the likelihood of accidents.
- Engaging in some type of exercise or body movement to promote rapid, appropriate movement of material through the intestines, and to improve muscle tone in the abdomen.
- Obtaining appropriate education about incontinence and fully exploring all avenues for treatment.

In sum, we should not allow our elderly patients suffering from incontinence to accept naively that their situation is hopeless (e.g., Slimmer, 1987). With the benefit of a trusting therapeutic relationship, we can encourage them to discuss their anxiety and fears in therapy. Talking about concerns with a romantic partner also can alleviate fears, and allow for "planned" bathroom breaks before romantic moments. We also can encourage our elderly male and female patients to seek medical and psychological consults for incontinence, for it can be treated in the majority of cases with up to an 80% success rate. Regarding different types of treatment, empirical evidence suggests that behavioral measures, such as biofeedback for pelvic muscle control and relaxation exercises during periods of increased urges to urinate, are significantly more effective at treating urge and mixed incontinence than are drug treatments (Burgio et al., 1998). Thus, mental health practitioners appear to be uniquely prepared to assist these patients.

## DEMENTIA

One of the most dreaded illnesses among elderly adults is that of dementia. Statistically, 10% of adults over the age of 65 are estimated to have Alzheimer's disease (Dorgan, 1995). Older adults may fear "losing their minds" and becoming a significant burden upon their elderly spouse or family members. Because a number of disorders can result in significant decline in mental status, including Parkinson's disease, vascular disease, Huntington's chorea, and Pick's disease, as well as Alzheimer's disease, a differential diagnosis becomes vital in coping with these debilitating disorders. Even though a relatively small number of older adults suffer from Alzheimer's disease (statistically), the life-altering course of the disease demands significant attention from geropsychological practitioners.

Caring for the Caregiver

A number of factors arise in consort with these dementing diseases in relation to sexual behavior. One of the most difficult problems often arises for caregivers who must redefine their role as both caregiver and spouse or lover (Ballard, 1995). The daily demands of caregiving can leave a caregiver feeling tired, anxious, and depressed. Tasks may range from helping their loved one to climb the stairs to helping their loved one use the toilet, bathe, dress, and eat. Caregivers have described this perceived change in role as distressing. One elderly woman described her transformation from spouse and lover to doting parent. She noted with disdain that after she "changed [her husband's] diapers and put on his bib to feed him," she felt too much like his mother to even consider kissing or cuddling him. It somehow felt safer for her to stroke his head and cheek, and literally pat him on the head as she often did with her sick children. It appears that ingrained incest taboos surface among caregivers who feel that they serve more of a parenting function, and thus could not possibly engage in an intimate, sexualized relationship with their spouse, who now effectively represents a childlike figure (Duffy, 1995).

Many caregivers report that their loved one has two deaths—the death of the personality or "true self" followed by the slow death of the body. Many caregivers feel that their intimate relationship ends when their spouse can no longer recognize them or know their name. Other caregivers report that they are too tired after physically demanding daily routines to even consider sexual contact. Still others describe anger and resentment interfering with any thought of a love life. One elderly gentleman responded by saying that he missed his wife's cooking and cleaning. He was forced to take a new role at home and although he knew it was not his wife's "fault" that she was ill, he was angry that he had to learn how to cook, do the laundry, shop for groceries, and clean the house. He said that he could not imagine having sex with a woman who was clearly no longer his "real wife." Certainly, it is not a therapist's place to encourage a caregiver to seek out sexual contact with a spouse with dementia. Rather, it is more helpful to caregivers to vent their frustrations and to articulate their perceived change in roles to manage their frustration and anxiety.

Changes in Sexual Behavior

In contrast, a small number of caregivers have reported an increase in sexual satisfaction and closeness with a partner who has dementia (e.g., Ballard, 1995; Duffy, 1995). Some described feeling closer to their spouse because they were engaging in a familiar, comforting activity that did not require words. Others mentioned that they liked the increased sexual attention from their spouse; one symptom of dementia is decreased impulse control, which may result in more frequent sexual advances. Still others felt that sexual behavior had a calming effect on their spouse, allowing both of them to relax and reduce overall levels of tension and stress in the household for a few hours. However, the vast majority of caregivers find such changes in sexual behavior puzzling and distressing (Duffy, 1995). A number of questions and concerns have been reported among elderly caregivers and these include:

- Anger and confusion when their otherwise caring, sensitive partner wishes to engage in intercourse without any foreplay. This apparently insensitive behavior is more likely to be a reflection of difficulties in remembering the correct "order" or sequencing of events (Duffy, 1995). Just as an elderly person with Alzheimer's disease may attempt to put on his pants before putting on his underwear, damage to the temporal lobe may result in such a person's attempt to engage in intercourse before emotionally and physically readying their partner. Sometimes redirecting a confused spouse can be effective. For other caregivers, the simple knowledge that this abrupt behavior is motivated by neurological deficits and not a disregard for their emotional needs can allay anxiety and upset.
- Fears that their partner may begin to expose him- or herself or engage in sexual behaviors in public. It is notable, however, that the majority of patients with Alzheimer's disease do not engage in public sexual displays (Duffy, 1995). If an elderly person with dementia does lift her dress or unzip his pants in public, it is more likely to be a sign of uncomfortable clothing or a need to toilet versus a sexual urge (Ballard, 1995).
- Distress that after a sexual liaison, their partner attempts to engage in sex again, as though forgetting what had just taken place. Similarly, anxiety has been reported among caregivers whose spouses became hypersexual as a result of their Alzheimer's disease (Duffy, 1995). These partners even described feeling frightened about the consequences (e.g., possible temper tantrums and angry outbursts) if they would not go along with their spouse's wishes for sex. Sometimes distraction and redirection are useful in these cases, but it is important to note that the underlying emotional distress caused by these incidents does not fade as quickly as the behavior is temporarily thwarted.
- A sense of duty to perform sexually for their partner, particularly among female spouses, even if they are emotionally unavailable or averse to the idea (Duffy, 1995). Many women from the current elderly cohort subscribe to the notion that they are to perform for their husbands both in the kitchen and in the bedroom; "a good wife never says 'no.'" A frank, objective discussion of this role within the context of a therapeutic rela-

tionship may help caregivers avoid the guilt associated with this belief and make a more appropriate assessment about whether they would like to engage in sexual relations with their disabled spouse or not.

• Fears that others in their caregiver support group will not understand their sexual concerns. One elderly woman noted, "Well, I just assumed that people would think I were a dirty old lady or that I was just selfish if I wanted to talk about sex with Gerald.... I love him and want to take care of him, but I just don't want to have sex with him now ... what will the other ladies think of me?" Because group therapy and support groups can be so vital for older caregivers, group leaders can initiate discussions about such sexual concerns in order to promote supportive group norms and to validate existing concerns among members.

It also is important to note that most research regarding the impact of dementing illness on sexual functioning focuses almost exclusively on men and women in the advanced stages of the illness. It is notable that in most clinical contexts, patients suspected of suffering from dementia are often ignored during clinical interviews and therapy trials. Even if a patient has some intact mental capabilities, the caregiver is attended to almost exclusively in terms of decision making and needs for therapy. It is as though it is so upsetting for both clinicians and family members that this patient was diagnosed with dementia, that the patient in question is ignored out of primitive attempts at denial.

Although challenging, involving both partners in therapy if a spouse is in the early stages of the illness can allow for a discussion of future plans for sexual relations as well as other future plans about long-term care, end-of-life issues, financial planning, and learning how to "say good-bye." One elderly man recently diagnosed with Alzheimer's disease said that he wanted that time to talk with his wife about his guilt for "leaving" her in the prime of their lives, to discuss ways to make the house safe for his grandchildren to come visit in case he forgot to turn off the stove, and to tell his wife about his love for her and the value he places on their marriage on both emotional and physical levels. Although this couple shed many tears in therapy, they resolved some important issues from their past and were better equipped to plan for the future. This gentleman's wife noted that she was able to enjoy their sex life until he no longer recognized her. "We both discussed that when he didn't know me anymore, it was all right to think he was gone.... I didn't have to feel guilty about saying 'no' to him after that.... I can now honor his memory and take care of him out of duty and love."


## PARKINSON'S DISEASE

Another chronic illness that affects up to 1 in 100 adults over the age of 60 is Parkinson's disease. In such individuals, the substantia niagra, a cortical structure in the midbrain, does not produce sufficient quantities of the neurotransmitter dopamine. The resulting lack of dopamine usually leads to classic symptom presentations of motor dysfunction. Some of these primary symptoms include a resting tremor of the extremities, difficulties in initiating movement, an overall slowing of movement, stiffness in the limbs, speaking in a low, raspy voice, and blank or masklike expressions. These motor disturbances certainly can impact on an older adult's sexual expression; one is less likely to feel "sexy" with a visible, potentially embarrassing resting tremor or a perceived inability to communicate with others. Older adults with Parkinson's disease also are at greater risk for developing dementia and depression than members of the general population (Knight, Godfrey, & Shelton, 1988), which also are known to interfere with elderly sexuality.

The drugs used to treat the symptoms of Parkinson's disease appear to have side effects that alter the sexual response cycle (see Cummings, 1991, for a review). On a positive note, L-dopa and Sinemet, the primary drugs used to treat Parkinson's disease, have been reported to restore prior interest in sexual activity, improve erectile function, and increase rates of masturbation, as well as to improve overall motor skills. However, these drugs also have been documented to induce hypersexuality (i.e., excessive masturbation that interferes with normal daily functioning, initiation of extramarital affairs if one's spouse does not consent to increasingly frequent sexual activity) or sexually deviant behavior— in up to 13% of patients. (Fortunately, these symptoms may be controlled in most cases by a reduction in medication or the addition of antipsychotic agents such as lithium.) Examples of observed deviant behaviors include self-injurious behavior, voyeurism, pedophilia, and exhibitionism. It also may be assumed that our patients are unaware of the sexual side effects often associated with their medication. Older adults with Parkinson's disease would benefit from intensive, interdisciplinary treatment from both psychological and medical practitioners in order to manage their illness successfully and to navigate changes in sexual interest or function.

## CHRONIC MENTAL ILLNESS

Managing chronic mental disorders such as schizophrenia and bipolar disorder can be challenging at any age. However, advanced age can make the treatment of such disorders even more difficult because of increasing concerns about side effects from medications, medical complications from other chronic ailments, and toxicity effects over time. At times, the presence of a serious infection or cancer may prevent elderly patients from taking their psychotropic medications, and may lead to an emergence or exacerbation of symptoms. Caregivers of these patients often are not asked how these disorders impact on their relationship or their sex lives.

The use of antipsychotic and mood-stabilizing medications alone can result in altered sexual function. The prescription drugs in Table 6 have been shown to produce side effects that can drastically alter the normal sexual response cycle. Side effects can range from a decrease in sexual interest to difficulties achieving orgasm (see Schiavi & Segraves, 1995).

TABLE 6.   Examples of Antipsychotic Medications
that Can Induce Sexual Dysfunction

| Drug name | Brand or trade name | Drug name | Brand or trade name |
| --- | --- | --- | --- |
| Lithium | Eskalith, Lithonate | Chlorpromazine | Thorazine |
| Haloperidol | Haldol | Mesoridazine | Serentil |
| Clozapine | Clozaril | Thioridazine | Mellaril |
| Trifluoperazine | Stelazine, Suprazine | | |

In the instance that a patient with a chronic mental illness suddenly is unable to take his or her medications, the resulting change in functioning can be extremely distressing and confusing to a romantic partner or spouse. Sexual acting out or sexualized delusions can be particularly difficult to cope with, for both patients' partners and their health care providers.

Paul

Paul was a 68-year-old man who came to a geropsychiatry outpatient clinic for treatment of depression. He was a quiet, religious man (of Catholic faith) with an obsessive character. His history revealed that he married at 26, and at that time he was aware that "something was wrong" with his wife. She would sometimes be too frightened to leave the house, and she had to quit her job as a receptionist. A few years later, she was diagnosed with paranoid schizophrenia. Paul said that he enjoyed his role as protector and provider; it made him feel like he was fulfilling his marital obligations and he felt competent because he managed most of the household chores while working full time as a mechanic. With the development of more effective psychotropic medications, Paul's wife became able to enjoy being a housewife and mother. She could tolerate going to church, cooking light meals, and participating in small social gatherings. The couple had four children, and Paul was delighted to follow his religious beliefs and bear children. It was one of his most important roles in life, next to being a faithful husband. Unfortunately, two of the couple's children were institutionalized in their mid-30s after developing paranoid schizophrenia.

In the past year, however, Paul felt that his wife was becoming more and more distant. He had researched her illness thoroughly, and felt that she was becoming increasingly paranoid. As had been the case early in their marriage, Paul's wife feared leaving their home and would sometimes scream out for no reason, or point to strangers and shudder in fear. Paul decided to seek help for himself for depression after his wife was diagnosed with bone cancer. Her chemotherapy and radiation treatments were difficult, and her physicians advised against her taking her psychotropic medication. A few months into her treatment for bone cancer, Paul's wife was diagnosed with inoperable brain cancer. Paul was overwhelmed with fear, anger, and grief.

Paul was most depressed about losing his life partner. They forged a bond over the years, and Paul was content in his role as advisor, protector, husband,

and lover. Although he gave limited details in therapy, Paul said that he always felt emotionally and physically close to his wife. He noted that when she was particularly upset (i.e., agitated or paranoid), sexual contact would calm both of them and "remind them of what life was really about." Although he was not able to articulate his position fully, Paul's feelings of inadequacy in his own family (he was seen as the "least capable" of 10 children) were negated when he took on the role of rescuer and potent husband in his own marriage to a woman with a chronic illness. Paul again began to feel inadequate as his wife's cancer metastasized. She began to lose control over her bladder and needed help feeding herself. When he could no longer take care of her daily needs at home, he placed her in a nursing home. He experienced this as a personal failure, and was upset that he could not provide for all of her needs.

Paul placed his wife's "needs" above his own, and his stoically obsessive character would not allow him to easily express his feelings of fear and loss. During one session, Paul's otherwise calm demeanor was shattered when he balled his hands into fists and shouted angrily, "Damn her illness! Damn it! I can't take it, just not this!" When asked what had happened, Paul's eyes began to water and his voice softened. He said that his wife's delusions had begun to change. Even though he knew logically that they were likely to be influenced by the growing tumor invading her brain, he still could not accept that "some part of her really thinks that!" During his last visit to the nursing home (Paul drove over one hour each way to visit her and did so almost every day), his wife recoiled from his touch. She screamed at Paul and said, "My husband is Jesus Christ! He is my husband!... Get out of my bed. He is my lover, my true lover! I want him in me now! Now!... Get away from me. God is my boyfriend ... who the hell are you? Get your hands off me.... You aren't holy!" Paul became suicidal when his wife said that God became her lover. His hands shook when he said plaintively, "I have given up my life to God and so, what, he, he takes my wife?! What did I do to deserve this?"

It took quite a bit of work in therapy for Paul to articulate his anger at God for allowing this terrible tragedy to happen, and for his wife to forsake him when he felt he was fulfilling his religious duty to serve her as a dutiful husband in sickness and health. Paul's suicidal ideation ceased when he was able to openly discuss his more "carnal" needs and his anger about being rejected by his wife, who for all ostensible purposes "should be thankful" for his love and patience. On some level, Paul could accept that her delusions may be, in part, an unconscious reflection of his deep religious beliefs and also a means through which his wife could distance herself from the relationship in order to avoid feeling the pain of their impending separation. When he was able to articulate his anger, face his repressed feelings of inadequacy, and acknowledge the bitter irony of his wife's choice of delusional lover, he became better able to reach out to others as well as to his wife. He rekindled friendships with men with whom he worked, his adult children who were living in other states, and a widowed male neighbor from across the street. Even though his wife could not understand what he was saying to her in her last days, Paul was able to tell her that he loved her and that he understood how she "could turn to God" so completely.

## SEQUELAE OF SEXUAL TRAUMA

Although not a chronic illness per se, the effects of sexual abuse or trauma are believed to include long term personality changes and stress responses such as posttraumatic stress disorder, borderline personality disorder (Davies & Frawley, 1994; Kroll, 1993), and psychosomatic illnesses. Although he later retracted it, Freud's original seduction theory posited that sexual trauma in childhood, particularly among young women, was repressed. These unconscious, repressed memories later emerged as hysterical neuroses (Freud, 1896), which could be described in current terminology as conversion hysteria and somatic disorders.

Along with anecdotal reports (e.g., Feil, 1995), recent empirical evidence derived primarily from studies of children and young adults suggests that sexual abuse such as rape and incest may be repressed (or poorly integrated or processed) to emerge later as somatic disorders (Bagley, Bolitho, & Bertrand, 1995; Bowman & Markland, 1996; Freedman, Rosenberg, & Schmaling, 1991; Friedrich & Schafer, 1995; Fry, Beard, Crisp, & McGuigan, 1997; Kinzl, Traweger, & Biebl, 1995). Young men and women with histories of abuse have been shown to have a greater likelihood of somatic, dissociative, and affective disorders (Bowman & Markland, 1996), and to exhibit specific somatic symptoms such as vocal cord paralysis (Freedman et al., 1991), vomiting, headaches, rashes, allergies (Friedrich & Schafer, 1995), suicidal gestures (Bagley et al., 1995), and painful intercourse among women (Fry et al., 1997; Kinzl et al., 1995).

Virtually no empirical evidence exists to suggest that early sexual abuse can lend itself to the development or continuation of such somatic disorders among older adults. However, anecdotal evidence (e.g., Feil, 1995) is building to suggest that older adults simply do not outgrow or simply forget about past sexual traumas. Some clinicians may not even inquire about early sexual abuse during initial interviews, and may assume out of denial or optimistic ignorance that "time heals all wounds." Unfortunately, this does not appear to be the case. Developmental issues associated with aging itself can complicate past issues of sexual abuse. For an older adult who has lost mobility and independence as a result of some chronic illness, this loss of control may allow previously repressed memories of being abused and "out of control" to surface. Repressed memories of abuse also may be compromised when an elderly person's mental status becomes impaired through either dementia or delirium. Because of cohort effects, older adults who experienced sexual assaults as children may have been told by frightened parents that "it never happened" or simply to "forget about it." Most elderly people grew up in a time when societal prohibitions warned against discussing sexual issues in general, much less about discussing sexual abuse among family members or friends.

### Barbara

Barbara was an 89-year-old woman who lived in an assisted living complex. She had been living in the community, but could no longer care for herself after an extensive hip reconstruction. A few weeks after arriving at the center, she presented with a variety of somatic symptoms including nausea, headaches, dizziness, ringing in her ears, and "flashes of light" in her eyes. Extensive medical workups revealed no underlying strokes, high blood pressure, or any other physical basis for her ailments. Barbara soon took to lying in bed for most of the day. She seemed to enjoy getting attention from the aides and physicians, and began to ring for assistance more and more often during the day, while becoming more and more removed from her peers. Barbara agreed to begin work in psychotherapy after her fifth medical consult revealed no underlying physical problems.

In therapy, Barbara only reluctantly discussed her hip surgery. She often avoided her therapist's questions about her quality of relationships, and engaged in little introspection. One afternoon, a large package arrived for Barbara at the center. Her therapist asked Barbara what arrived for her, and she replied that it was a selection of new clothes in response to her distaste for her current clothing. Barbara had become upset when she was forced to wear a "frumpy" hospital gown and was ushered into bed by young orderlies or "hoodlums" after her surgery. She currently was very upset about her declining appearance, and began to spend a significant amount of time talking about feeling trapped in her bed, her wheelchair, and her room. When asked if she ever felt trapped before, Barbara started to cry, but would not respond directly to her therapist's gentle inquiry.

After working together for a few months, Barbara began to engage in scheduled social events at her extended care facility. She told her therapist that she took pride in her appearance, and that a decent-looking man asked her to go for ice cream together later in the week. When asked what she thought about this man, Barbara's voice became high-pitched and loud, "The hell with him, honey. Take them for all they're worth, that's what I say.... Who cares about him?" A discussion of her past relationships revealed that Barbara had been divorced twice, and that her husbands had always been furious with her constant flirting, batting of eyelashes, and wearing of dresses "cut up to there." Barbara told many stories about going out to fancy parties wearing scantily cut dresses, and getting men to take her to the finest restaurants and theaters. When asked if she wanted to settle down, she said, "That's all part of the game—to make them pay, you know? I could get their attention, that's for sure. A nice dinner, all the right gifts, but oh, no, you don't."

When asked what "oh, no, you don't" meant, Barbara said that that was "her power." When her therapist responded that she wanted to understand exactly what Barbara meant, she became frustrated and retorted, "Oh, my power, my power over all of them now.... I got my way back at them." Further discussion allowed Barbara to recount an incident that occurred when she was 18 years old. She had graduated from high school and took a job as a file clerk for a large trucking company. One afternoon, she ventured into the large garage looking for some old files. She had become friendly with some of the workers there (who were all men except for her and the boss's wife who only occasionally came to the office to help file things), and she felt comfortable asking them to move one of the large filing cabinets blocking some others in the corner. Barbara described that "out of nowhere," one of the guys grabbed her and said, "I'll help you, little lady." He pushed her into a back room of the trucking bay and raped her. He then called one of his buddies into the room and he raped Barbara, too. Barbara said that she had tried to scream, but they held their hands over her mouth and threatened to stab her with some "sharp-looking tools."

After the rape, Barbara got dressed, and went back to her desk, dazed. One of the truckers who befriended her saw her disheveled appearance and asked her what happened. Barbara said that she just sat there and shook her head and began to cry; "I couldn't tell him anything, not that, it was so horrible and I was so ashamed." The trucker apparently put two and two together, and went out into the trucking bay. He gathered up some other employees from the office, and apparently they discovered the two rapists and beat them savagely, requiring them to make a trip to the hospital. After this happened, Barbara said that "everybody was sure nice to me," but that nothing was ever mentioned about the incident. Barbara said that she went to the hospital a few weeks later for "a nervous breakdown," and that her boss came to visit her and offered her a retirement package, even though she had only worked there for a few months. Barbara took the retirement package and left town shortly after to live with her aunt.

A few months later, Barbara married the first man who showed any romantic interest in her. He was a member of a minority group, and her family took the news of the marriage badly. She said that her husband became "understandably frustrated" with her because she found sex with him painful and anxiety provoking. (She made no connection between her rape and her stunted sexual relationship with her husband.) Her husband became even more "frustrated" when Barbara began to buy and wear sexy clothes and to flirt openly with other men, even when they were "out on the town" together. The marriage ended a year later when her husband asked for a divorce. Barbara moved into an apartment with a co-worker from the local phone company, and began "moving up the social scene" by targeting successful men for flirtation. She always made sure that she had very limited time alone with her dates, and often ended a relationship "before it really got started." Her second marriage to a wealthy businessman ended when he had an affair with his secretary, who Barbara assumed was "more free in bed."

The breakup of her second marriage put Barbara into "second gear." She resumed her flirting and socializing with vigor, and recognized that her anger at men could best be engaged by employing her feminine wiles. As she became older, however, she became increasingly "sick." As her appearance deteriorated, related in part to her adult years of heavy smoking and drinking, Barbara found that she could not get the kind of "male attention" that she was used to. Her headaches, dizziness, and muscle aches worsened, and she became a frequent visitor to various physicians' offices and hospital clinics. By the time she arrived at the assisted living community, she herself felt that she had little hope to "get anything from men anymore," and had begun to garner male attention exclusively through her psychosomatic symptoms. After she was able to discuss her rape in therapy, Barbara's symptoms subsided somewhat. Barbara noted that "even after all of these years," she did not realize how "fresh" those memories were when she talked about them. With each telling of her story, her anxiety level diminished, and she was able to accept that it was not her fault in any way, and that she had nothing to be ashamed about. Barbara went on to develop some meaningful same- and opposite-sex friendships in the assisted living community.

## SUMMARY

A number of challenges face many older adults who suffer from chronic mental and physical illnesses, as well as acute psychological and physical disorders. A variety of ailments themselves, such as Parkinson's and Alzheimer's disease, can impinge upon an older adult's sexual functioning directly. Sometimes the treatment can be as detrimental as the disorder itself in terms of sexual functioning. For example, the medications commonly used to treat certain illnesses including high blood pressure, diabetes, arthritis, and schizophrenia can alter an older adult's sexual response cycle. Other disorders, such as urinary incontinence, can be effectively treated with conservative measures, and most members of the public as well as members of the mental health community are unaware of these recent advances. Other aspects of a person's life, such as the experience of early sexual trauma or disfiguring surgeries such as mastectomies in later life, have the potential to impact negatively on older adults' sex lives. In many cases, the caregivers of elderly patients require as much attention as the elderly patients themselves. Thus, it has become increasingly vital for clinicians to become knowledgeable about various illnesses that become more common with age, and about how both their course and treatment can impact on their elderly patients' and their caregivers' sexual expression.

# 6

# HIV/AIDS among Older Adults

*The oldest person to have a documented case of HIV infection was an 88-year-old white widow. She is believed to have been exposed to the AIDS virus through sexual contact with her husband, a recreational intravenous drug user (Rosenzweig & Fillit, 1992).*

Health care providers can no longer afford to regard HIV and AIDS as a disease of youth and young adulthood. According to the Centers for Disease Control (CDC, 1995), more than 11% of all new AIDS cases in the United States occur among men and women over the age of 50. Seven percent of these cases are reported among men and women over the age of 60, who may be considered young-old, and 4% of all of these reported AIDS cases are among men and women over the age of 70, who may be considered elderly. In the past few years, more older adults have contracted HIV than have adults under the age of 30. Between 1990 and 1992, the number of new AIDS cases among young adults decreased more than 3%, while the number of new AIDS cases among older adults (over the age of 60) increased more than 17%. Specific areas of the country in which older adults have increased in number, such as Florida, California, and Arizona, also report substantial increases in numbers of AIDS cases among older adults. In Palm Beach County, Florida, approximately one half of all new AIDS cases were among adults aged 50 and over. AIDS is now the 15th leading cause of death among men and women over the age of 65 (Kaye & Markus, 1997). Some estimates suggest that by the end of the century, more older adults will die of AIDS than the number of Americans killed in the Vietnam War (McCormick & Wood, 1992).

Additionally, CDC statistics may underestimate the actual numbers of infected persons in the older adult age group because of underreporting (e.g., family members often ask that their physician identify a non-AIDS cause of death on their relative's death certificate), misdiagnosis, and the exclusion of older adults who may be asymptomatic except for the cognitive changes associated with HIV induced dementia. Ageism, particularly regarding negative stereotypes and misconceptions about elderly sexuality, appears to reduce the ability of health care providers to gather vital patient information, and to make and report accurate diagnoses. A reluctance of practitioners to discuss an older adult's participation in high-risk behaviors also hinders appropriate diagnostic assessment.

The implications for such an incorrect or a delayed diagnosis of HIV among older adult patients are insidious. Such clinical errors can postpone the delivery of appropriate medical, psychological, and psychosocial interventions, and can ultimately result in increased patient mortality, along with a decrease in overall quality of life (Linsk, 1994). Because of a decrease in immune system functioning, older adults who contract HIV are likely to die sooner than their younger counterparts, even if both persons were diagnosed and treated at the same time. Malpractice suits against health professionals are another likely outcome that may occur when delayed and inaccurate diagnoses of HIV infection are made among older adult patients.

## TRANSMISSION OF HIV

### Identifying Risk Factors

Epidemiologists expect that by the next century, more than 10% of all AIDS cases will be among adults aged 60 and older (McCormick & Wood, 1992). This expected growth in numbers is related to increases in heterosexual transmission of the virus in the middle-aged and older adult age groups, typical decreases in immune system functioning with age, and the longevity of people living with HIV and AIDS (Catania et al., 1989). The modes of transmission of HIV among older adults are somewhat different than those among younger adults. For middle-aged and older adults over the age of 50, the most likely means of viral transmission are:

1. Homosexual male contact (62% of all cases)
2. Intravenous drug use (11%)
3. Heterosexual contact (10%)
4. Blood transfusions (8%)
5. Use of blood clotting products by hemophiliacs (1%)
6. Caregiving for HIV-infected children (<1%)

Approximately 8% of all AIDS cases among older adults have an unknown or unidentified means of transmission.

The rates of transmission among heterosexual men and women are expected to increase into the next century as a more sexually active younger age cohort comes of age. At the same time, the number of AIDS cases associated with tainted blood transfusions (administered primarily before 1985) is expected to plummet as a result of increased safeguards in our blood supplies. Older adults have been at greater risk than younger adults for contracting HIV through blood transfusions, reflecting the fact that an older adult is more likely to require lengthy operations that are more likely to require transfusions such as knee and hip replacements, open heart surgeries, and exploratory surgeries to correct internal bleeding after an automobile accident.

It also is notable that nearly one tenth of all AIDS cases among older adults have not been traced to a specific high-risk group or high-risk behavior. It is unclear whether these cases are unaccounted for because health care providers are reluctant to document that their elderly patient engaged in a high-risk behavior, or whether medical personnel simply were unable to identify the source of the infection because of lack of appropriate information gathering. For example, although infection with HIV has been reported among elderly parent caregivers of adult children with AIDS, and more than one third of all people with AIDS rely on their parents for daily care (Allers, 1990) very few official reports of such transmission have been made by the CDC. In one case, AIDS was believed to be contracted by exposure to infected bodily fluids during an elderly mother's caregiving activities ("HIV transmission in household settings," 1994). This 75-year-old woman said that she often forgot to wear gloves when she came in contact with her son's bodily fluids.

To illustrate another example of a potentially overlooked risk factor for HIV infection among elderly adults, the case report of the oldest individual diagnosed with AIDS was an 88-year-old white woman who purportedly contracted the virus through sexual intercourse with her husband, a recreational intravenous drug user (Rosenzweig & Fillit, 1992). What is most intriguing about this case is that this women was a widow; she was diagnosed with AIDS 7 years after the death of her husband. It took a bit of detective work, careful risk assessment, and sensitive questioning by very open minded clinicians to arrive at the appropriate diagnosis, and to deliver the appropriate treatment.

Risk Factors Specific to Older Adults

Older adults have more high-risk factors for contracting AIDS than once believed. Increased age itself does not prevent older adults from engaging in intravenous drug use or unprotected heterosexual and homosexual contact. Despite common stereotypes and misconceptions, older adults have been shown to engage in heterosexual and homosexual activity into late life with relatively high frequency, and have been found to frequent prostitutes of both sexes, just as adults from younger age groups do. The use of illicit substances also has been increasing among older adults, including the use of intravenous drugs such as heroine and cocaine. It is vital that clinicians address such issues in their initial diagnostic interview.

Women and men over the age of 50 are significantly less likely to use condoms than their younger counterparts, particularly when a female partner is postmenopausal (Linsk, 1994). When asked about their use of condoms during sexual relations, some of my patients have laughed and responded, "Oh, my. You know that I don't have to worry about a baby on the way! But that is flattering that you would think about me being so young to even ask. You are so sweet." Other patients have responded to questions about condom use with some variant of, "Oh, that's just for people who are dirty, you know what I mean?

My Reggie and I have been together for over a year. I don't have to worry about anything. He's squeaky clean." Men are more likely than women to influence whether a condom will be used during sexual intercourse, and older adult males are the least likely age group to use a condom. Most older adult patients I have talked to do not even consider heterosexual contact as a risk factor for HIV, particularly if they are widow and widower who assume that their partner had been involved in a long-term monogamous relationship. Older adults can be just as easily lulled as clinicians into the false belief that AIDS is an "evil disease" that is only a problem for young people.

Postmenopausal women who engage in vaginal intercourse are at increased risk for contracting HIV. Because of a variety of hormonal changes, the resulting decrease in vaginal size and lubrication are more likely to lead to microscopic and macroscopic vaginal tears during intercourse, which provides easier entry for the virus into the bloodstream (Catania et al., 1989). Like most younger adult women, the majority of older adult women are not even aware that sexual intercourse is often accompanied by such trauma to the vaginal wall because these tears are often painless and generally undetectable after intercourse. Coupled with the general decrease in immune system functioning with age, an increased risk of vaginal trauma, and overall lower rates of condom use, an older adult woman has a higher risk of contracting HIV through each act of heterosexual intercourse than her younger adult, female counterpart.

## A NEED FOR PREVENTION STRATEGIES AND EDUCATION

To make matters worse, older adults are less likely to be targeted for HIV prevention strategies, and are less likely to be knowledgeable about the nature, transmission, and progress of the disease (Allers, 1990; Solomon, 1996). Older adults are less likely to be cognizant of the 4- to 7-year "window" that may pass between initial infection with HIV and the emergence of symptoms. Thus, they may be more likely to unknowingly pass the virus to their partners and loved ones through sexual contact and intravenous drug use (Catania et al., 1989). Few educational programs about HIV and its transmission exist for older adults or for health care providers. Although some cities have developed extensive AIDS education and outreach programs, virtually none have delivered their important message to sexually active older adults. Among health care providers, only a handful of training programs in academic and on-the-job settings incorporate geriatric issues, much less specific issues about HIV among older adults, into their required curriculum.

## KNOWLEDGE AMONG CAREGIVERS AND PRACTITIONERS

To date, only one attempt has been made to explore health care providers' knowledge and attitudes about HIV among older adults (Hillman, 1998). Employing a sample of psychiatrists, psychologists, and nursing personnel at a large mental health facility that featured numerous, specialized geriatric units, the results showed that these health care workers correctly identified homosexual men and women, and intravenous drug users as among the top two risk groups for HIV transmission among adults over the age of 50. However, although a significant number of the health care workers in the study were aware of the increase in HIV transmission among heterosexual older adults, the vast majority were not aware of the increased risk of HIV transmission via intercourse in post menopausal women. They estimated that an older adult woman who was date raped by an HIV-infected rapist had the same chance of contracting HIV as a young adult woman raped by the same assailant. The clinicians also misidentified elderly recipients of blood products as being at lower overall risk of contracting the virus than documented by the CDC.

It is notable that in all risk groups except for heterosexual men and women, at least one participant incorrectly maintained that *no* individuals over the age of 50 in certain risk groups, including intravenous drug users, sexually active homosexual males, and caregivers of adult children with AIDS, were at risk for contracting HIV. It is as though these participants maintained the stereotype that elderly adults simply do not engage in certain high-risk behaviors, and that older adults are mercifully immune from danger when caring for an adult child infected with HIV. The health care practitioners also were unaware of the appropriate treatments available for older adults who are suffering from AIDS and HIV induced dementia.

Contrary to expectation, exposure to various patient populations including adults over the ages of 50 and 70, and exposure to patients who have HIV was not associated with more accurate knowledge of HIV and its transmission among older adults. Also contrary to expectation, specialized training in HIV, geriatrics, neuropsychology, and human sexuality was not associated with greater knowledge. It is unclear whether the specialized training that these health care providers received broached the subject of HIV. However anecdotal, after the study was over, a number of participants remarked that they had never even considered that an older patient of theirs might have HIV, and that they had never received any formal or informal education about it. It is clear that as clinicians, we must correctly educate ourselves and our patients.

## ASSESSMENT AMONG OLDER ADULT PATIENTS

### Questions at Intake

Ageism exists when health care providers fail to ask, or even consider, whether their older adult patients are at risk for contracting the AIDS virus. To make an accurate diagnosis, it is vital that clinicians ask their older adult patients candidly and directly about a variety of issues including (see Hillman & Stricker, 1998, for a review):

- Sexual history (including extramarital affairs and multiple partners)
- Current sexual behaviors (including vaginal, oral, and anal intercourse)

- Recreational drug use (particularly intravenous drug use)
- Major operations and blood transfusions (especially before 1985)
- Use of blood products for hemophilia (especially before 1985)
- Caregiving for AIDS patients
- Sexual abuse or assault
- Changes in mental status such as apathy and confusion
- Physical symptoms such as swollen glands, loss of appetite, and a nagging cough or cold

Health care providers should never assume that an elderly patient is free from the risk factors associated with HIV transmission. The potential emotional discomfort associated with asking elders about their sexual activities and sexual history is well worth the effort if it reveals a possible link to an HIV diagnosis and to timely, appropriate treatment. It also is vital that clinicians remember that a 4- to 7-year window often passes between infection with the virus and overt symptoms. Thus, sexual history remains a vital part of any intake assessment, regardless of a patient's age, marital status, or current sexual abstinence. Recall that the oldest patient to have a documented case of HIV infection was an 88-year-old woman who had been widowed and sexually abstinent for more than 7 years.

We know that older adults, as well as younger adults, use intravenous drugs, have affairs, employ prostitutes, and become victims of sexual assault. It also is important to ask older adults if they have had more than one partner in sexual relations, and if they have had partners of the same or different sex. Another salient item for questioning regards caregiving activities for patients with AIDS, particularly with adult children who may be living at home and receiving total nursing care from an elderly parent. Although these topics certainly can be difficult subjects to broach, the information to be gained is invaluable.

The Presence of Family Members

Because of the sensitive and private nature of these questions, it may be advisable to speak to an older adult patient without the spouse, significant other, or children being present for the entire interview. For better or worse, many older adult patients come to an initial interview with a spouse, a caregiver, and children. Additional information from family members can provide important information that might otherwise be lost, and their presence allows the clinician to observe family dynamics firsthand. However, it often is advisable to discuss at the beginning of the interview that some time will be allotted to speak to the designated patient alone. Many patients become noticeably more relaxed about the procedure when they are told that it simply is standard procedure to do so.

It also can be helpful to preface questions about a patient's sexual history and high risk behaviors by telling him or her that these are standard questions asked of every single patient at every single interview. It is important to inform patients that whatever information they discuss with you is confidential, and that this information will not be disclosed to other family members without their expressed, informed consent, with the exception of mandatory reporting for danger to self or other, and elder abuse as prescribed in some states. Normalizing the discussion of such typically private matters as sexual behavior and drug use often allows patients to speak freely and to express additional concerns (e.g., Hillman & Stricker, 1998). It is important that clinicians use the same sexual terms as the ones used by their patients. If an older adult woman feels more comfortable talking about her lover's "sex organ" than his penis, follow her lead. Of course, if a patient begins to use language that a clinician finds particularly vulgar or degrading, it is appropriate to resort to general anatomical terms.

## The Benefits of a Team Approach

Regardless of the clinician's degree status, professional title, or proscribed role on a treatment team, each mental health professional should take personal responsibility to ensure that a potential HIV diagnosis is examined and, ideally, ruled out. The use of a team approach can provide a professional cohort to discuss and work through any feelings of discomfort regarding the discussion of high-risk behaviors and potential HIV status with a patient. Just as we often inform patients that we often have little control over how we feel, but that we are responsible for how we manage those feelings, it is vital that team members remain respectful of others' feelings, even if they appear negative, ambivalent, or anxious. However, once such feelings have been aired and processed within the group dynamic, team members typically are better able to manage those feelings appropriately so that they do not interfere with the assessment and treatment of patients. Often the team member who has the most rapport with the patient, or the team member who has the greatest comfort with discussions about sexuality can play the role of mediator and patient educator, with favorable results.

## The Importance of Follow-Up

Even after assessment takes place, it remains vital that clinicians remember that older adults are the least likely group to be targeted for educational interventions regarding HIV and its transmission. In most cases, patient education is as important as proper assessment. Despite ageist stereotypes, patients of all ages should be educated about having protected sex. Among older adults, particularly those who may have postmenopausal female partners or who have same-sex partners, the fear of conception is absent. Thus, this older age group is least likely to use "safe sex" because their associations to such measures are solely for pregnancy prevention. Older adults may not even know how to use a condom properly. Elderly intravenous drug users also may not be aware of the use of bleach and the avoidance of needle sharing to minimize the transmission of HIV. Older adults also are not likely to be aware of universal health precautions. Such information is critical, particularly when an older adult provides one-on-one nursing care for an adult child infected with AIDS.

Marsha

Marsha was a 68-year-old woman enrolled in a geriatric day hospital program. Marsha was admitted on the recommendation of her adult daughter who was concerned that no one was available to help her mother manage her obsessive–compulsive disorder and keep up with her activities of daily living. Marsha's daughter is her only child from her first marriage, which ended more than 20 years ago in divorce. Marsha arrived on time each day for the program, and was always dressed and groomed neatly for someone of her size. Marsha reports that she gained over 75 pounds in the last 5 years; she is obese. She also appeared to demonstrate some difficulties with attention and concentration.

Although she agreed readily to participate in group psychotherapy, Marsha had significant difficulty avoiding her compulsions, even under the influence of appropriate medication. During group sessions, she would only be able to sit for a few minutes at a time before she would feel compelled to walk seven steps forward, three steps backward, turn 180 degrees, and repeat the procedure in varying degrees. She also whispered to herself as she counted numbers in a complicated pattern. It initially was unclear how much Marsha would benefit from the day program's group therapy and milieu therapy because of the severity of her symptoms. Her daughter reported that they intensified about 5 years ago, when she also changed her eating habits and began to gain a significant amount of weight. Neither Marsha nor her daughter could identify a precipitating incident.

Three months into the program, Marsha experienced a breakthrough. She had begun to socialize with two elderly single women who had also been secretaries who enjoyed big band music. Marsha began to eat lunch with these women and to be able to stave off some of her compulsions long enough to talk with them in brief conversation. During a group therapy session, one of these women discussed how vulnerable she often feels in her own home, because her late husband is no longer there to look after her. Marsha, who had been whispering to herself, gave her new companion a sideways glance and began to rock back and forth and hum loudly. The group leader paused to ask Marsha how she was doing, and Marsha began to cry. She admitted that about 5 years ago, a maintenance man she had hired to do some chores around the house suddenly became violent and raped her. She swore that she would never tell anyone about the attack because she felt so ashamed and afraid. Marsha received overwhelming support from other group members, and was able to discuss the event more openly over the next few weeks. She learned that it was not her fault about what happened, and that it was normal for her to feel angry, embarrassed, and upset. Marsha also was able to explore the relationship between her desire to control her environment via her compulsions and her attempts to feel comforted and reassured with the consumption of food.

Despite the positive response that Marsha received in group therapy among her elderly peers, the treatment team did not demonstrate such cohesion when Marsha's group therapist suggested that Marsha be informed about the risks of contracting HIV and other sexually transmitted diseases, and to assist her in scheduling an AIDS test. The initial response among team members was that it was just "water under the bridge." Marsha's individual therapist asserted that she did not want to broach the subject of HIV testing because it would only retraumatize her patient, and lead to a resurgence of binging and compulsive behavior. After all, this happened more than 5 years ago!

A lengthy discussion ensued in which many team members were able to discuss their anger and discomfort about the thought of a gentle and innocent older woman contracting HIV through a senseless and violent acquaintance rape. When the team leader asked how they would proceed if Marsha were a 25-year-old woman who had been raped, they quickly recognized their conscious and unconscious desires to deny the entire unfortunate incident. Many of the team members also acknowledged their implicitly held stereotype that "well, elderly women just don't get AIDS." In a parallel process like that observed in the patients' group therapy session, in which group members were able to rally around Marsha after she aired her secret about the rape, the treatment team was then able to support Marsha's group therapist in her need to discuss the issue openly. The team agreed that it was vital to speak sensitively but frankly with Marsha about the rape and about her subsequent risks for contracting HIV. Because one of the nurses on staff had a particularly good relationship with Marsha, she volunteered to meet with her to address specific medical questions and the hospital's policy regarding HIV test results.

### Gerald

Gerald was an 83-year-old man who was brought to the geriatric assessment unit of a hospital after having a serious fall at home. Concerned neighbors in the apartment complex called the police when they had not seen Gerald for a few days. Gerald appeared malnourished and unkempt, and he presented with a low grade fever and swollen glands. On admission he was confused and apathetic when staff members tried to communicate with him. He preferred to spend his time on the unit alone, curled up on his bed. After being contacted by the staff social worker, Gerald's estranged son agreed to go to his father's apartment to gather his pajamas and toiletries. While at his father's apartment, Gerald's son discovered a large collection of empty liquor bottles, and vials of white and brown powder. The treatment team concluded that Gerald was suffering from major depression and substance abuse, and suggested that he enroll in an inpatient treatment program for drug abuse. The team physician ordered a series of chest x-rays and considered using antibiotics to treat a probable case of pneumonia. The treatment team did not even consider HIV as a possible diagnosis, even when Gerald admitted to intravenous drug use.

## OLDER ADULTS AS CAREGIVERS

### Demographics

Just as many older adult grandparents are assuming the role of caregiver for their grandchildren, many older adult parents are assuming the role of caregiver for their adult children who suffer from AIDS. With the increasing number of AIDS patients in this country, difficulties with medical insurance coverage, an inability to acquire hospital or hospice care, and a lack of other available caregivers, many elderly parents, particularly elderly mothers, are providing daily nursing caring for adult children dying of AIDS. Some elderly parents describe having a positive experience, in which they are able to show their children that they love them, even to the bitter end. Other elderly patients in this caregiving role have spoken to me about acknowledging and accepting their child's homosexual lifestyle for the first time, and about forgiving their child for turning to drugs as a way to deal with their problems. Other elderly patients have been more reluctant caregivers, and have voiced concerns about who will care for them when they are sick and in need of caregiving. Still other caregivers have discussed how preoccupied they are with keeping the nature of their child's illness a secret from friends and family members. They fear that no one will visit them or want to socialize with them after their child has passed away.

Florence

Florence was a 75-year-old widow who exhibited symptoms of depression and dementia. Her niece insisted that she enroll in a day hospital program in order to help lift her spirits, and Florence reluctantly agreed. Florence arrives at the day program each day, dressed appropriately and neatly. She is eager to make friends with other patients in the program, and quickly acquires a close-knit circle of five female companions for breakfast, lunch, and conversation between group sessions. During group therapy, Florence is eager to participate. She responds supportively to patients dealing with a variety of problems, yet can also gently challenge their denials and cognitive distortions. Before long, most patients in the day program clamor to sit with Florence, to hear her tell a humorous story or to offer a kind word. Although Florence is reluctant to discuss her own problems in group therapy, her depression appears to lift, and her mood brightens. She tells the group that she has been doing more cleaning and baking at home. She even brings a loaf of her special apple bread to share with her group of friends.

About 1 month into the program, it became obvious that Florence was having trouble remembering things. She often forgot to take her hat home, or forgot to bring an umbrella when it was raining. She sometimes lost track of what people were saying in group therapy, but could use her sense of humor to smooth over any rough spots. Her primary therapist asked for a neuropsychology consultation to rule out dementia, and Florence agreed to participate. The neuropsychology intern said that Florence was superficially cooperative, but that she became very frustrated when she couldn't trace a series of lines, remember a series of words, or recite parts of a story. The official report suggested that Florence had mild to moderate dementia, with unknown etiology; the pattern was not entirely consistent with Alzheimer's or vascular dementia. The test report also contained suggestions that Florence use a notepad to help remind her about daily medications and physicians' appointments, and that she be retested within 6 months to see if she would benefit from instrumental assistance around the house. Florence did not take the news well, and insisted that, of course, she forgot things once in a while, but that she was "as fit as a fiddle."

About 2 months into the program, Florence failed to arrive on time for the morning session. Because she had not called in sick, her primary therapist called her home, and initially thought she had dialed a wrong number because a younger woman answered the phone. The therapist was surprised because Florence had told her that she was a widow of more than 15 years who lived alone. The woman on the phone said that she was Florence's daughter, and that Florence was taking a little longer than usual to help her with her morning routine. Florence herself refused to discuss the issue over the telephone, and said that she would come to the program at the regular time on the following day only if her therapist promised that they would discuss the issue "in private."

When asked about her situation at home, Florence admitted that her daughter was dying of AIDS. She implored her therapist to keep it a secret from the other patients, and only reluctantly accepted that this information would be shared (in confidence) among the treatment team members, as per the usual agreement for acceptance into the program. Florence said that it was her duty as a mother to take care of her daughter, but that things were very difficult for her. When asked why she never talked about this serious problem behavior, she said that she didn't want to burden others with her problems or "waste time crying over spilled milk." Despite her therapist's urging, Florence felt strongly that there was no need to discuss this problem with others in group therapy, because it would probably just make others upset.

Although she never had formal nursing training, Florence was proud that she learned how to help her daughter with her catheter, change her dressings (she apparently had open wounds that were not properly healed), and help her eat, bathe, and go to the bathroom. She said that she was faring much better with this daughter than with her son, who died of AIDS 5 years previously, also under her care. When asked how her two children contracted the virus, Florence tersely replied that they had turned to "dirty street drugs." Although Florence never provided a wealth of details, it also appears likely that her daughter turned to prostitution to finance her drug habit, and that she could have contracted HIV through unprotected heterosexual sex. Florence failed to mention whether or not she wore latex gloves and goggles when taking care of her daughter and son, or that she even knew how to properly dispose of potentially contaminated medical waste.

Within the treatment team, concerns were raised that Florence was not even aware of the basic universal precautions required for caring for someone with AIDS, and that even if universal precautions were explained to her, her dementia would prevent her from employing them accurately and consistently. However, the treatment team was reluctant to discuss universal precautions with Florence, much less ask her to consider an HIV test for herself. Some staff members admitted openly that the topic of AIDS made them uncomfortable, and that they simply did not want to "put Florence through that with everything else she has been through." Staff members also argued about whether Florence should be encouraged to discuss her situation with her peers. Many staff members expressed fear that the older adults in the program would ostracize her and even engage in a mass exodus from the program in order to avoid contracting the disease. Heated discussions also arose about whether staff members and patients alike should take universal precautions when dealing with Florence on a daily basis. Ultimately, Florence agreed to have a visiting nurse help with some of her daughter's caregiving. She refused to take an HIV test, and never disclosed to her peers that her daughter had AIDS.

### Universal Precautions

What are the appropriate universal precautions for an older adult parent caring for an HIV infected child? The U.S. Environmental Protection Agency suggests the following:

- Gloves and other barriers such as goggles must be used every time contact may be made with bodily secretions.
- Remember that bodily secretions can be encountered through feeding, bathing, adjusting catheters, dressing wounds, and providing mouth care.
- Hands should be washed with soap and water after gloves are removed.
- Needles, lancets, and syringes should be disposed of in metal containers that can be sealed, such as coffee cans secured with heavy-duty tape.
- Soiled bandages, sheets, and gloves should be placed in sealed plastic bags before being thrown out with other trash.
- If the HIV-infected patient has tuberculosis, caregivers should keep the area well ventilated and receive periodic skin testing.

### Protection for the Practitioner

Health care providers must observe universal health precautions with patients of all ages, including our older adult patients. These patients include the pleasant 88-year-old widow who arrives for treatment of an infected insect bite that just won't heal, as well as the verbally abusive, 25-year-old intravenous drug user who arrives for treatment for a rare type of pneumonia. Of course, these patient examples are generalizations and stereotypes in themselves. However, it is vital that health care providers learn that HIV does not spare anyone of illness, whether they are young or old, "sweet" or "nasty," or wealthy or indigent. As health care providers, we must learn to protect ourselves as well our patients.

## HIV-INDUCED DEMENTIA

### Symptom Presentation

Like its older cousin, syphilis, HIV has been found to cause significant neuropsychological problems that often present in the form of dementia. Autopsy studies suggest that up to 80% of individuals who contract AIDS will develop HIV-associated dementia complex (HADC; American Academy of Neurology AIDS Task Force, 1991). Clinical studies also suggest that more than one-third of all people currently infected with HIV will meet diagnostic criteria for dementia (Buckingham & Van Gorp, 1988). Recognizing the causal relationship between such a sexually transmitted disease and a debilitating dementia is particularly important among older adults, whose symptom presentations of HADC may mimic, and subsequently be mistaken for, Alzheimer's disease.

A number of researchers have provided comprehensive summaries of the symptoms associated with HIV induced dementia (Lipton & Gendelman, 1995; Mapou & Law, 1994). These symptoms include, but are not limited to, cognitive symptoms such as impaired attention, impaired concentration, poor short-term memory, confusion, and impaired abstract thinking; affective symptoms such as apathy, indifference, and social withdrawal; and behavioral symptoms such as psychomotor slowing, diminished coordination, unsteady gait, difficulty with writing, impaired occupational functioning, and a significantly decreased ability to engage in activities of daily living. It is important to note that unlike Alzheimer's dementia, HADC typically includes both cognitive and psychomotor impairment. The American Academy of Neurology AIDS Task Force (1991) also identifies HIV Associated Minor Cognitive/Motor Disorder as a neurological syndrome in which an individual infected with HIV does not yet meet criteria for dementia, but exhibits mildly or moderately impaired functioning.

### Differential Diagnosis with Alzheimer's Disease

Practitioners must be aware that the symptoms of HADC often mimic the classic symptoms of Alzheimer's disease. Table 7 summarizes the similarities and differences typically observed in their symptom presentations. Both disorders present with a debilitating picture, in which patients display significantly diminished social and occupational functioning, and short- and long-term memory loss. However, some vital distinctions can be made between the typical presentations of HADC and Alzheimer's dementia. Regarding onset, HADC tends to be sudden, whereas recognizable onset of Alzheimer's dementia typically is gradual. HIV-induced dementia often has a rapid, aggressive progression over a period of 6 months to 1 year, whereas Alzheimer's dementia has a gradual progression of symptoms, often over many years. Language impairment, such as aphasia (an inability to speak), is not a part of the typical HADC presentation, unlike the typical presentation of Alzheimer's dementia. No pronounced language deficits are observed in HADC, until the very end stages of its progression.

Although short-term memory is significantly impaired in both HADC and Alzheimer's dementia, patients with HIV-induced dementia, unlike their counterparts with Alzheimer's dementia, appear to maintain their ability to encode (or learn) new information. For example, although most patients with HADC and Alzheimer's dementia display impairment in their recall of a list of words, even after numerous repetitions, the patient with HADC would be more likely to recognize certain words as part of the original list (indicating that she or he was

TABLE 7.   Differences betwen HIV-Associated
Dementia Complex and Alzheimer's Dementia[a]

| Symptoms | HIV dementia complex | Alzheimer's dementia |
|---|---|---|
| Onset | Acute | Gradual |
| Progression | Rapid | Gradual |
| Time until acute stage | 6 months–1 year | More than 1 year |
| Affect | Appropriate | Labile |
| Mood | Apathy, depression, mania | Depression |
| Psychomotor speed | Significant impairment | Minor impairment |
| Gait | Impaired | Intact |
| Use of language | Intact | Impaired (aphasia) |
| Short-term memory | Impaired | Impaired |
| Encoding | Intact | Impaired |
| Opportunistic infections | Common | Rare |
| Cerebrospinal fluid | Elevated protein levels | Average |
| T-cell count | Below average | Average |

[a]These characteristics represent a summary of typical symptoms. Each case of dementia is unique, and deviations from the typical symptom presentation must be expected.

able to encode the new information, but was unable to retrieve it without cuing). Patients with HADC, as compared to Alzheimer's disease, also appear to have significant impairment in psychomotor speed. When asked to connect thought with action, a patient with HADC is expected to display significant difficulty. Additionally, patients with HADC often display other symptoms of AIDS, such as low grade fevers, depressed mood, skin lesions, opportunistic infections (e.g., pneumonia, shingles), diarrhea, headache, night sweats, sudden weight loss, reduced sex drive, and incontinence. Clinicians should recognize that such symptoms, particularly those including reduced sex drive, depressed mood, memory impairment, and incontinence, are *not* a normal part of healthy aging, and should be explored as a sign of underlying pathology.

## POSSIBLE TREATMENTS

Although there is no cure for HIV infection itself, proactive treatment for older adults typically incorporates the use of antiviral agents such as azido-thymidine. Consistent monitoring with a caring physician is vital to maintaining a high quality of life and to decreasing patient mortality. Because an older adult's immune system may already be compromised by aging, it is vital that treatment begin as soon as possible after diagnosis. Recent research also suggests that the specific impairments associated with HADC may be minimized with appropriate treatment. Specific treatments for HIV-induced dementia include antiviral agents (Wallace, Paauw, & Spach, 1993), nitroglycerin (Lipton, Choi, & Pan, 1993), and psychostimulants (Holmes, Fernandez, & Levy, 1989). The use of support groups and psychotherapy can be an essential and effective part of treatment for elderly patients who have been diagnosed with HIV (Kornhaber & Malone, 1996), or who provide caregiving for an adult child suffering from HIV (Levine-Perkell, 1996). The names, addresses, and phone numbers of a variety of organizations that can assist older adults in dealing with HIV and AIDS are provided in the appendix at the conclusion of this chapter.

## SUMMARY

The rise in documented AIDS cases among older adults is unprecedented. The rates of infection are increasing nearly four times faster among older adults than among young adults. The primary means of infection among older adults include homosexual contact, heterosexual contact, and intravenous drug use. Despite the wealth of information that we now have about HIV among older adults, it is unclear how many older adults currently suffering from HIV and HADC remain undiagnosed and untreated. It also remains unknown how well-equipped clinicians are to make differential diagnoses regarding HADC and Alzheimer's dementia. Practitioners must guard against falling victim to their own ageist beliefs and stereotypes; dealing with older adults and HIV is a daunting but necessary task. The development of educational programs, and of subsequent outcome studies are some of the first proactive steps we can take to guard against ageist and inappropriate diagnostic decision making. An essential weapon against the inaccurate diagnoses of HIV and HADC is available through both practitioner and patient education.

## APPENDIX

Available Resources for Older Adults Dealing with HIV and AIDS

**American Association of Retired Persons (AARP)**
601 East Street NW
Washington, DC 20049
(202) 434-2260

AARP has a Social Outreach and Support (SOS) division that provides links to various referral services.

**HIV/AIDS in Aging Task Force**
425 East 25th Street
New York, NY 10010
(212) 481-7670

This task force arranges educational seminars and conferences for health care providers.

**National AIDS Clearinghouse**
P.O. Box 6003
Rockville, MD 20850
1-800-458-5231

This organization provides information about local resources and offers access to free government publications.

**National AIDS Hotline**
1-800-342-AIDS
1-800-344-SIDA for Spanish
1-800-AIDS-889 (TTY)

This hotline is manned 24 hours a day, 7 days a week. It can provide referrals to local programs and general information about the disease.

**Seniors in a Gay Environment (SAGE)**
305 7th Avenue, 16th Floor
New York, NY 10001
(212) 741-2247

SAGE offers referral services and HIV/AIDS information to gay and lesbian older adults, primarily in the New York metropolitan area.

**Social Security Administration**
1-800-SSA-1213

Social Security provides two different disability programs for eligible AIDS patients.

# 7

# Women's Issues
# in Elderly Sexuality

*Nearly one-third of elderly women report experiencing pain or discomfort during sexual intercourse. This is not, and should not be, considered "normal."*

Elderly women are often faced with contradictory messages about their sexuality. Many segments of our society, and particularly those from the media, practically insist that women remain beautiful, youthful, wrinkle free, physically fit, and sexually vigorous late into life. In contrast, other segments of the population espouse that older women should accept their role as passive, unassuming, amorphous, gender-neutral figures who would not even attempt to engage in sexual activity. Both of these directives conflict greatly with many elderly women's individual realities. In order to assist these elderly women in managing issues regarding their own sexual identity, it often is necessary to provide them with concrete information about the underlying physical changes that accompany normal aging as well as to explore parallel psychological and psychosocial issues.

## PHYSIOLOGICAL CHANGES

Empirical studies of the oldest-old segment of our population (aged 80 and older) suggest that men are two times more likely than women to engage in sexual activity such as sexual intercourse (Bretschneider & McCoy, 1988). Arguments have been made that a significant amount of variance in this relationship reflects the lack of availability of a partner for elderly women (Meston, 1997) and the persisting gender differences in patterns of sexual behavior that appeared in adolescence (Meston, Trapnell, & Gorzalka, 1996). However, older women have been found to engage in a variety of sexual behaviors, both with and without a male partner, that include more than coitus (Ludeman, 1981).

Because women's sexual activity also appears to be relatively constant through-out the life span (e.g., Janus & Janus, 1993), it may be more beneficial for clinicians to focus on an elderly woman's expectations and desires for sexual activity than any observed statistical differences between her rate of behavior and that of her elderly male counterpart.

Unfortunately, more positive attitudes toward elderly sexuality do not auto-matically translate directly into greater sexual expression among aging women. If an elderly woman wants to engage in greater sexual activity with her partner but experiences pain during intercourse, for example, she must be made aware of the underlying physical changes that accompany aging (and ways to mitigate such changes) in order for her to fulfill her increased sexual desire. Other women may be concerned that certain bodily changes they have been experienc-ing are "abnormal," and a sign of mental weakness or a loss of femininity. Be-cause of a general lack of information (e.g., Jones, 1994), such physical changes caused by aging are often misinterpreted or misunderstood by both elderly women and their health care practitioners alike.

## Menopause

Most physiological changes related to sexual function and aging in women begin somewhat abruptly with the onset of menopause, at approximately age 50 (Barile, 1997). Although certain symptoms such as hot flashes and headache have been suggested as culture or individual specific (but as equally valid and distressing; Barile, 1997; Robinson, 1996), other symptoms of menopause appear to be biologically universal. (Because this chapter is dedicated to a discussion of elderly sexuality, the more acute symptoms of early menopause such as hot flashes will not be discussed here as they are experienced primarily in midlife.) During menopause, the production of the hormones estrogen and progesterone decreases, while the production of follicle-stimulating and luteinizing hor-mones (FSH and LH, respectively) increases in an attempt to promote estrogen production. What this increase in FSH and LH actually tends to produce is an increase in testosterone, and some women are more likely to produce more or less of this hormone than others (Barbach, 1996). Some estrogen is produced in the body through the conversion of remaining adrenal androgens (Roughan, Kaiser, & Morley, 1993).

During this alteration in hormone production, the size of the uterus, cervix, and ovaries is reduced in response to the body's shifting of resources away from needs for reproduction; conception is no longer biologically possible (Zeiss, Delmonico, Zeiss, & Dornbrand, 1991). The uterus itself may be reduced in size, via changes in collagen and elastic content, by up to 50% (Woessner, 1963). Related to other changes that may be more directly apparent in sexual function, decreases in estrogen levels can result in a thinning of the vaginal lining, a loss of vaginal elasticity, and a decrease in vaginal lubrication (Barbach, 1996).

Sometimes, patients have described situations for which clinicians tell them that menopause is "all in their heads," and that their symptoms are motivated primarily by emotionality. In contrast, other women have complained that even though they have positive feelings about aging and their bodies, they feel like failures because they have allowed themselves to "fall victim" to menopausal symptoms of one variety or another. They assume that a positive mental attitude will prevent them from experiencing any biological changes or physical symptoms. Although some symptoms of menopause appear to be mediated by individual, societal, and cultural expectations (Barile, 1997; Robinson, 1996), a number of concrete physical changes do occur at this developmental milestone, and every woman's unique experience should be validated. Accordingly, it is vital for both patients and their practitioners to recognize that despite a postmenopausal woman's positive feelings about sexuality and high levels of emotional readiness and arousal, sexual intercourse may be experienced as painful and unpleasant without the use of appropriate interventions.

Adrenopause

Although a wealth of information has become available about menopause, significantly less is known about adrenopause, the further reduction in the production of adrenal androgen that begins at approximately age 65 among women (Roughan et al., 1993). With a reduction in adrenal androgen, even less hormonal estrogen becomes available as it had been produced peripherally through conversion of this androgen. Although it is unclear to what extent adrenal androgen plays a role in mediating sexual expression directly, recent studies suggest that while levels of androgen are not directly correlated with the frequency of sexual activity in women, higher levels of androgen are associated with a greater sense of well-being in women (Cawood & Bancroft, 1996; Morales, Nolan, Nelson, & Yen, 1994), which in turn is associated with sexual expression (Cawood & Bancroft, 1996). Some trials of androgen replacement therapy have been attempted with young-old women, revealing ambiguous results at best. In addition, some researchers warn that in high doses, androgen replacement therapy could cause side effects such as the emergence of facial hair, deepening of the voice, and liver damage (Barbach, 1996). Thus, empirical support is unclear regarding the usefulness of adrenal androgen replacement therapy among elderly women (Roughan et al., 1993) Perhaps more importantly for mental health care professionals, it remains unclear to what extent the experience of adrenopause may artificially decrease an elderly woman's sexual desire or expression.

Sexual Response Cycle

Some researchers suggest that once concerns about conception are alleviated by menopause, elderly women may find greater enjoyment in their sex lives. They are no longer saddled with beliefs that they must produce something in relation to sex, and sexual activity becomes pleasurable for its own sake (Koster, 1991). Others assert that our society views menopause as a medical disorder or deficiency, with negative expectations for social status, rather than as a normal developmental phase signifying greater freedom and an opportunity to reaffirm or redefine roles (Carolan, 1994; George, 1996; Robinson, 1996). Many American women may miss out on the opportunity to view menopause as a positive step in their lives, with accompanying sexual pleasure and expression. Nevertheless, many elderly women can expect that physiological changes related to aging can result in some alteration in their sexual response cycle, if not their actual enjoyment of sex. Understanding the typical changes that take place in sexual arousal may help elderly women and their partners adapt and enjoy sexual activity in spite of these changes.

The sexual response cycle can be categorized in four stages: (1) the excitement, (2) plateau, (3) orgasm, and (4) resolution stages. A variety of estrogen- and nonestrogen-related changes can impact on an elderly woman's response to sexual arousal. Refer to Table 8 for an overview.

One of the most obvious changes in sexual response with advanced age (in response to a decrease in estrogen production) is the reduction in quantity of vaginal lubrication. The majority of elderly woman also find that it takes significantly longer for them to become lubricated. While it once took only a few seconds to become "wet" or aroused by her partner, producing even inadequate levels of lubrication may now take well over a few minutes. In addition to experiencing painful intercourse as a result, an elderly woman may mistakenly assume that she is no longer feminine, or may misinterpret her lack of lubrication as an emotional cue that she somehow is no longer interested in her partner. In a parallel fashion, a male partner may feel inadequate because he requires more time to get his partner "ready," or he may feel upset or even angry that she requires more foreplay. He also may feel that he is no longer sexy or appealing to

TABLE 8.   The Elderly Woman's Sexual Response Cycle

| Stage | Age-related changes |
| --- | --- |
| Excitement | |
|   Vaginal lubrication | Delayed (may take up to 5 minutes versus 10–15 seconds among young adults) |
| | Reduced in quantity |
|   Vasocongestion | Reduced |
| Plateau | |
|   Uterine elevation | Reduced |
|   Labia majora | Reduced elevation |
|   Breast changes | Less vasocongestion |
| | Diminished nipple erection |
|   Clitoral stimulation | Maintained or heightened, sometimes producing irritation |
| Orgasm | |
|   Vaginal contractions | 2–3 contractions (between 5 and 10 contractions among young adults) |
|   Uterine contractions | Weaker and shorter in duration |
|   Subjective experience | Pleasurable sensations maintained |
| Resolution | |
|   Capacity for orgasm | Maintain potential for multiple orgasms |
|   Vasocongestion | Rapid loss and return to prearousal state |

his partner, particularly if he feels anxious or ambivalent about his own advanced age. In contrast, sometimes increased skin sensitivity makes breast, nipple, and clitoral stimulation irritating instead of arousing (Galindo & Kaiser, 1995). In a worst-case scenario, an elderly woman does not inform her partner that she simply needs more time and additional lubrication in order to mutually enjoy sexual relations. Such painful intercourse (i.e., postcoital cystitis or dyspareunia) may be accompanied by vaginal bleeding, burning sensations, and swelling both during and after sex (Bachmann, 1995). These women may suffer in silence out of shame and misunderstanding as well as out of a poor sense of entitlement related to dependent personality traits.

An elderly women, and her partner, also may be pleased to learn that her subjective experience of arousal may be just as strong and pleasurable as that experienced by her younger female counterparts. Pleasure from stimulation of the breasts remains intact, despite a lesser likelihood of vasocongestion and nipple erection (Kaiser, 1996; Roughan et al., 1993). And, despite changes in the objective experience of orgasm—an older woman is likely to experience more shallow, less frequent vaginal and uterine contractions (Leiblum & Rosen, 1989; Zeiss et al., 1991)—the overall subjective experience of orgasm as pleasurable remains virtually unaffected by age. Elderly women also remain capable of experiencing multiple orgasms within the context of one sexual encounter (Leiblum & Rosen, 1989). In sum, it appears that advanced age may have the most detrimental effect during the excitement or arousal stage of the sexual response cycle. However, once an elderly woman becomes adequately aroused and lubricated (either naturally or with assistance), she can expect to experience subjective sexual pleasure and satisfaction consistent with that experienced by women many years her junior. The other physiological caveat is that once an older woman experiences orgasm, her body refracts rapidly to her prearousal state. Care and time must be taken to reestablish proper arousal and lubrication before additional acts are attempted.

## CLINICAL ASSESSMENT

The proper assessment of an elderly woman's sexuality and sexual functioning is vital. Mental health care providers often serve as indirect or direct liaisons between elderly female patients and their physicians or other physical health care providers. Sometimes an elderly woman may feel more comfortable discussing sexual issues with a therapist with whom she has developed a long-term relationship than with a gynecologist whom she visits once a year. Alternatively, physicians may refer elderly patients to a psychologist or other mental health practitioner in response to concerns over sexual dysfunction that were revealed in an introductory interview. (Of course, out of respect for a patient and in deference to ethical and legal issues, the patient's consent must be obtained in order to share even cursory information between professionals.) Psychologists must be attuned to appropriate modes of assessment, and also to general medical knowledge that may illuminate aspects of sexual dysfunction.

Dangers of Incomplete Assessment

Estimates suggest that up to 30% of middle-aged and elderly women experience pain during intercourse (Bachmann, 1988). Individual research studies suggest that older women experience an increase in discomfort and a decrease in sexual pleasure with advancing age (Thirlaway, Fallowfield, & Cuzick, 1996). Although such pain can certainly be associated with medical disorders such as skin lesions or cysts, such dyspareunia often is caused by atrophy of the vagina coupled with inadequate lubrication during intercourse. Mistakes in making such a determination have led to serious consequences for elderly women. Anecdotal reports suggest that elderly women who reported having vaginal bleeding after intercourse underwent cystoscopies and D&C's under general anesthesia simply because their practitioner assumed that these elderly women were not sexually active, and because they did not even inquire about their current participation in sexual activity (Butler et al., 1994). Many elderly women themselves, particularly because their cohort has not been well educated about sexuality, do not recognize that vaginal bleeding and inflammation may be their body's natural response to painful sexual intercourse without appropriate lubrication.

Specific Areas of Inquiry

A variety of pointed questions may be asked when working with an elderly female patient who has concerns about her sexual health and activity. As with any patient, it is important that practitioners tell their patients that being open and honest will allow for the greatest benefit to them. Older patients also often respond well to being *asked* if they would mind answering questions about their sexuality. This asking of permission provides an elderly patient with some sense of control over a potentially anxiety-provoking situation, and also provides for an established sense of commitment regarding her cooperation during the interview. If an elderly woman defers from discussing her sexuality, it is best to respect her decision, but to inform her that you are open to a discussion of such important issues with her at any time in the future (Galindo & Kaiser, 1995). It also can be helpful to retort, "I respect your decision not to discuss matters of sex with you, and will not ask you any questions about it as you wish. However, I do wonder if you *would* be willing to share with me *why* you decided not to talk about it at this time." Confidentiality and rules about sharing (or the lack of sharing) of information with team members of other professionals also are essential in order to provide a safe environment and to delineate professional boundaries for the patient.

Depending on your familiarity with the patient, use terminology consistent with her experience. If you are meeting with a patient for the first time, it often is helpful to use medical terminology but to then shift to the vernacular as required. Some of these questions can be adapted to a paper-and-pencil format, where patients are instructed to check off concerns and items for future discussion. In individual interviews, it often is helpful to preface sensitive questions with an initial assessment of the older woman's religious prohibitions, marital or partner status. Certain subsequent questions could be tailored to accommodate the elderly patient's specific situations or concerns (Kennedy, Hague, & Zarankow, 1997). Examples of assessment questions that address specific issues related to female elderly sexuality (e.g., Galindo & Kaiser, 1995; Kennedy et al., 1997) include:

- What kinds of sexual activity do you engage in? (Offer a variety of options such as hand holding, hugging, kissing, bathing, massaging, fondling, oral sex, finger penetration, vaginal intercourse, anal intercourse, masturbation.)
- How important is sexual activity to you in your life?
- Would you like to engage in more or less sexual activity?
- If you would like to engage in more sexual activity, what do you think is keeping you from doing so? Are you tired, ill, without a partner, is your partner tired or ill, have you lost interest, are there relationship problems, are you worried about what people will think, do you have religious concerns?
- Do you experience pain or discomfort during penetration or while having sex?
- Do you have vaginal pain or dryness, either before or during sex?
- Do you experience bleeding during or after sexual intercourse?
- Have you considered using a lubricant during sex such as KY jelly or Vaseline? (Vaseline is not an appropriate choice for vaginal lubrication because it is oil based, but many elderly adults use it because it is readily available.)
- Have you ever experienced orgasm with your partner? Has that changed at any time in the past few years?
- How often do you masturbate or touch yourself to feel good?
- How often do you have the urge to have sex? Is this different than from before? In what way?
- Have you or any of your partners had sex with anyone who used intravenous drugs, visited prostitutes, or engaged in homosexual relations? (Allows for an assessment of high risk behaviors.)
- Has anyone ever forced you to have sexual relations that you did not want to have? Has anyone ever touched parts of your body when you did not want them to? (Be sure that the patient knows that this includes historical as well as recent events.)
- How do you feel about your appearance? About your body? Have you had any surgeries that have changed either the appearance of your body or how it works, such as a mastectomy or colostomy?
- How are your eating habits? Are you concerned about your weight? Do you ever binge, purge, or use laxatives to control your weight?
- When is the last time you were seen by a gynecologist or had a pelvic exam? What is it like for you when you go to the gynecologist?
- When is the last time you had a pap smear? Have you ever had cervical cancer or an abnormal pap smear? Do you have a family history of cervical or ovarian cancer?

- When is the last time you had a breast exam or mammogram? Have you ever had breast cancer or cysts? Do you have a family history of these illnesses?
- What questions, if any, do you have for me regarding sexual function or behavior?
- Do you have any chronic illnesses such as diabetes, arthritis, or depression? How does that affect how you feel about yourself and your body?
- Are you currently taking any prescription or over-the-counter medication?
- Do you exercise or meditate?

It is often challenging to ask any patient, much less an elderly woman if she has engaged in high-risk sexual behavior. It is our obligation as clinicians to search for the truth, and not make any age biased assumptions about our elderly female patients. Straightforward but diplomatic wording of such questions is vital. For example, when trying to assess whether an elderly woman's partner visited prostitutes, one might ask matter of factly, "Do you think that your spouse was always faithful?" The less anxious the interviewer appears about potentially sensitive topics, the less anxious the older adult patient will be in response. With elderly women in particular, it is as essential to assess issues regarding subjective body image as well as issues regarding objective frequencies of sexual behavior and breast cancer screenings. Sometimes simply asking an elderly woman about whether she has difficulty finding clothing that she likes may bring up issues of shame regarding a mastectomy or difficulties in feeling attractive regarding a dowager's hump.

## SIDE EFFECTS OF MEDICATION

Although discussed less in the literature, older women are just as likely as older men to experience negative, sexual side effects from various prescription and over-the-counter medications. Some discrepancies in reporting may reflect the more objective, easily observable criteria related to male sexual function (i.e., the maintenance of an erection). The female sexual response is more difficult to measure empirically and generally relies on older women's subjective experiences, which have been generally overlooked by researchers in the past. Table 9 presents a variety of drugs that are believed to disrupt the female sexual response cycle, fostering inadequate vaginal lubrication, a decrease in libido, and the inability to achieve orgasm. Women who take these drugs should be advised to consult with their physician if they are concurrently experiencing sexual discomfort or problems.

## MITIGATING PROBLEMS

Although many sexual problems among elderly women stem from a combination of psychological, relational, and psychosocial causes (Butler et al., 1994; Chrisler & Ghiz, 1993), physical changes with age can underlie and compound

TABLE 9.   Medications that May Induce
Negative Sexual Side Effects in Older Women[a]

| Medication class | Drug | Generic or brand name |
| --- | --- | --- |
| Antidepressants | Clomipramine | Anafranil |
| | Fluoxetine | Prozac |
| | Imipramine | Tofranil |
| | Paroxetine | Paxil |
| | Sertraline | Zoloft |
| Antihypertensives | Clonidine | Catapres |
| | Chlorothiazide | Diuril |
| | Digoxin | Lanoxin |
| | Prazosin | Minipress |
| | Reserpine | Diupres |
| Antipsychotics | Chlorpromazine | Thorazine |
| | Clozapine | Clozaril |
| | Haloperidol | Haldol |
| | Thioridazine | Mellaril |
| | Trifluoperazine | Stelazine |
| Chemotherapy agents | Various | |
| Mood stabilizers | Lithium | Lithonate, Eskalith |

[a]This listing is not comprehensive; a variety of other medications may elicit similar
  side effects.

many existing problems. Fortunately, some means are available in assisting elderly women and their partners in mitigating many of the hormonally induced changes that occur with aging. Many of the remedies employed are designed to combat the loss of estrogen.

Topical Lubricants

One of the most easily employed treatments to deal with the vaginal dryness that often accompanies aging is the use of supplemental lubrication. A topical, water based lubricant, such as Astroglide or KY jelly, is recommended. These products are easily obtained without a prescription, at any local drug store, and they do not carry a risk of side effects. Many elderly women assume that Vaseline petroleum jelly or a moisturizing hand or skin cream will serve a similar purpose. However, Vaseline is not advised because it is oil based, and not easily absorbed into the skin. Such oil-based products also erode latex condoms, the only means of preventing sexually transmitted diseases. Even though elderly women are not concerned about unwanted pregnancies, they should be aware that sexually transmitted diseases are not reserved only for the young. Similarly, moisturizing hand lotions may be oil based or may contain a variety of dyes and perfumes that can cause skin irritation and infection.

It is important to recognize the psychological implications of using an "aid" in sexual intercourse at any age. Although it appears an easy solution to employ such topical lubricants during sexual intercourse, many elderly women may be uncomfortable applying them in front of their partner before intercourse, or they may feel embarrassed or inadequate because they need to use them. Communication between an elderly woman and her partner is essential in order for both parties to feel comfortable using such lubricants. They sometimes can be incorporated into intercourse as foreplay, which also benefits the older woman who has a physiologically induced slower arousal phase. For women who opt not to use water-based lubricants immediately before intercourse, other alternatives have been offered. These include over-the-counter products such as Replens or vitamin E oil (from capsules) applied vaginally on an alternate day schedule (Barbach, 1996).

Masturbation

Masturbation is another effective, nonhormonal treatment for vaginal dryness that often comes as a surprise to both elderly patients and their practitioners alike. Women who remain sexually active, either through sexual intercourse with a partner or through self-stimulation, have been shown to show a lesser decrease in vaginal lubrication with age (Roughan et al., 1993). Although the exact mechanism is unknown, it is posited that masturbation increases blood flow to the vaginal area, which promotes increased lubrication on a daily basis (Galindo & Kaiser, 1995). Because of numerous religious and societal prohibitions against masturbation, suggestions to engage in self-stimulation must be discussed sensitively, particularly with older patients. Respect for an elderly woman's religious prohibitions against masturbation must take highest priority, and should circumvent any further discussion of the issue.

In contrast, some women who are burdened by social taboos about masturbation feel liberated when the practice is "prescribed" by their psychologist or other health care provider (Galindo & Kaiser, 1995). Anecdotal evidence suggests that some female patients have been cured of insomnia, vaginal dryness, and symptoms of anxiety after being instructed by their clinicians to experiment with masturbation before bedtime. Elderly women also may be encouraged to learn that masturbation does not necessarily involve penetration into the vagina with a finger or a foreign object. Manual stimulation of the clitoris and labia is often enough to induce sensations of pleasure, orgasm, and the desired increase in blood flow.

Hormone Replacement Therapy

Physicians often prescribe estrogen replacement therapy to assist older women in dealing with the physiological changes induced by a lack of hormonal estrogen. Estrogen replacement therapy has been touted as effective in combating vaginal atrophy and dryness, reducing the risk of heart attack, stroke, and heart disease, reducing the risk of osteoporosis and subsequent bone fractures, and decreasing the incidence of insomnia (Belchetz, 1994). More ambiguous claims exist regarding estrogen's potential to enhance sex drive (Belchetz, 1994) and to defer the onset of dementia (Kampen & Sherwin, 1994) and depression in late life (Palinkas & Barrett-Connor, 1992). Some counterindications for estrogen replacement therapy include breast cancer, fibrocystic breast disease, liver disease, unexplained vaginal bleeding, and endometriosis (Petrovitch, Masaki, & Rodriguez, 1996). What remains central for most mental health practitioners is not, however, whether our elderly female patients are prescribed estrogen replacement therapy or not. What is important is our ability to help our patients communicate openly with their physicians in order to make the choice that is most appropriate for them (e.g., Paganini-Hill & Henderson, 1994).

## CHANGES IN SEXUAL SELF-CONCEPT

In American society, women typically are judged on their physical appearance. Despite unrealistic expectations from the media and other sources to remain in a state of perpetual youth, women can naturally expect to experience changes in their body's shape and appearance as they age (Chrisler & Ghiz, 1993). As well as inciting changes in internal organ structure and vaginal lubrication, menopause is believed to initiate changes in a woman's distribution of body fat, and thus induce changes in her overall appearance. Specifically, women tend to gain weight at the onset of menopause (Rodin, Silberstein, & Streigel-Moore, 1984), resulting in an average body fat composition of 46% compared to an average premenopausal percentage of body fat of 23%. As adrenopause approaches, the average woman's percentage of body fat can be expected to reach 55% (Rodin et al., 1984). Additionally, locations of body fat storage may be redistributed to the breasts, waist, and upper back (Voda, Christy, & Morgan, 1991), which may change some women's physiques and even require them to find different clothing to accommodate their body's changing shape (e.g., Jackson & O'Neal, 1982).

Other, more general physical changes associated with normal aging impact on an elderly woman's appearance and her experience of sexuality. As noted, our society equates youth with sexuality; an elderly woman in particular must navigate difficult issues involving both her own attitudes toward her body's changes and society's general disdain for the aging female body, which should be swaddled in discrete clothing and cloaked in restorative creams and makeup (Chrisler & Ghiz, 1993). Empirical studies suggest that at all ages, women, as compared to men, manifest greater concern about their body shape and weight, and that they maintain significantly lower self-esteem in relation to their appearance (Pliner, Chaiken, & Flett, 1990). At an extreme, some elderly women have expressed concerns that young children may find their aging faces and bodies "scary" (Bernstein, 1990). How women interpret and internalize these changes greatly influences their sense of self and subsequent expressions of sexuality and sensuality.

### Identity Issues for Women with and without Partners

For some elderly women, body image is a central construct, a core feature of their identity that gives them pause for consideration on a daily (or in some cases, an hourly) basis. These women's daily experience of their aging body may serve as a narcissistic injury to their previous sense of self, or inner object world, which relied heavily on an outwardly youthful countenance. Accordingly, when a sample of elderly women were asked about their body image in relation to their sexuality and sensuality, the vast majority cited that they were concerned about their energy level, physical health, and nutritional status. Most flatly denied that they had any concerns about their sexual identity; in fact, most responded that it simply was not really a consideration "at my age." However, the vast majority of these women also expressed significant interest in wearing fashionable makeup, clothing, and wigs, belying their interest and apparent pleasure, concern, and pride that they took in their appearance (Campbell & Huff, 1995).

In contrast, other elderly women view their body's appearance and function as less central to their identity. These women view their femininity and inherent worth as less of a reflection of their external appearance, but rather as a function of their satisfaction in personal relationships, their personal accomplishments, and sense of spirituality. Empirical studies also have suggested that women who feel that they have greater control over their lives, who place less importance on arbitrary standards of physical attractiveness, and who feel positive about their worth as human beings have a more positive body image (Rackley, Warren, & Bird, 1988). Thus, an internal locus of control appears beneficial for an elderly woman, particularly regarding her sense of acceptance and mastery over her health, appearance, and body image.

For many elderly women, even for those who reported satisfaction with their appearance, issues of body image may become particularly salient after the death of a spouse or long term partner (Malatesta et al., 1988; Porcino, 1985). After mourning the partner's death, a renewed sense of urgency may occupy her thoughts as she prepares to enter the dating scene and faces the pervasive double standard that submits that women, but not men, gain access to new romantic partners primarily as a function of their appearance. Other elderly women find that once their lifelong partner is no longer available as a sexual partner (e.g., either through death or because of personality and physical changes as a result of advanced dementia), their interest in maintaining a sexual identity is equally diminished. For the vast majority of women, however, concerns about one's appearance persist throughout life, and these concerns originate from both internal (e.g., desires to feel feminine and attractive) and external sources (e.g., social pressures to be attractive to gain acceptance). Clinicians can often provide elderly women with the permission that society does not grant them to address these sexually related pleasures, fears, and anxieties, whether they are with or without a romantic partner.

Margaret

A number of elderly women participated regularly in group therapy for caregivers. Each woman's husband was seriously ill, and required significant nursing demands. Nearly all of the patients concurred that the greatest difficulty they had in their new role of caregiver was that they felt that they had little time or energy for themselves. For many of these group members, the hour spent in group therapy was one of the only activities they engaged in that focused on their own needs and interests. During one session, Margaret mentioned that while she accepted with some measure of pride that the marriage vows she took included loving and caring for her husband "in sickness and in health," she missed his arms about her at night and their intimate moments together. (Her husband was in the end stages of Alzheimer's disease and he remained virtually motionless in a hospital bed.) The other group members then collectively discussed their loss of interest in sex and sensuality. One group member quipped, "Who has time for that anymore, anyway? I'm lucky if I can get out to come here, or to run to the store to buy some groceries." Others debated about whether their sex lives really were that important anymore, "since [we] are older and we don't have husbands to be with that way anymore, anyway."

In response, the therapist made a direct request for each woman to buy and use scented body lotion when bathing and getting dressed in the morning. When some of the women balked at this homework assignment, stating that they did not have time for something so "silly," the therapist reminded them that they could easily purchase such products at the local drug or grocery store, or even by mail order in a cosmetics catalogue. She encouraged them to humor her and "give the activity a try," and then make their individual decision about how they felt about it. She also encouraged the group members to sample a variety of products and to select the fragrance that they liked best. She also directed them to allow themselves an extra few minutes in the morning to rub the lotion on their legs, stomach, chest, and arms as they got dressed.

During the next week's session, Margaret and a few other women in the group actually brought their scented bath oils and lotions with them to the group to show each other. Margaret said that she initially felt guilty about taking the time to go shopping and buy herself something, but that she began to feel better once she got home and used her lotion. "It is as though it follows me throughout the day ... it reminds me about the group, too, when I start to feel down." Other women said that they had not paid much attention to different parts of their bodies in a long time, and that "it wasn't as bad as I thought; my stomach isn't that big after all." Another woman said, "I hadn't been in the make-up aisle in a long time. I bought myself some new blush, too." She was able to acknowledge that she still received pleasure from tending to her appearance and "feeling feminine," even though she had not done so in a long time because of her involvement in caregiving. Still other women reported that the use of the lotions allowed them to acknowledge and mourn their personal losses, "I had forgotten how Sam used to help me with my lotion on my back. I miss his touch on my skin.... It makes me sad, yes, but it also makes me remember.... And now I can do some of that for myself.... I'm still a woman, too, even if my husband can't hold me anymore."

In sum, these women renewed their interest in their bodies and in basic sensual pleasures. The therapist's "prescription" for the use of perfume and scented oils allowed these women to explore and begin to focus on their own bodies. Many were pleasantly surprised to renew their own sexual identities, without direct input or feedback from their husbands. As caregivers, they had been granted permission to tend to themselves.

## AGE-RELATED CONCERNS IN BODY IMAGE

Although it is obvious that elderly women have concerns about their body image as do their younger counterparts, the specific concerns and anxieties that elderly women have are likely to be very different from those held by their juniors. The following have been identified as common concerns related to body image among elderly women:

- Facial changes (wrinkles, age spots, sagging chins)
- Graying and thinning hair
- Gnarled hands caused by arthritis (both for appearance sake and for the resulting lack of mobility to get dressed, groom oneself, and engage in tactile stimulation of self or partner)
- Incontinence (including fears of odor and dislike for the baggy, loose clothing sometimes required to accommodate large pads)
- Poor posture and gait resulting from arthritis, hip replacements, or other ailments
- Dowager's hump caused by osteoporosis (postural concerns and difficulties with finding attractive clothing)
- Impaired vision (may reduce ability to ambulate and to groom oneself)
- Hearing loss (making it difficult to communicate and socialize)
- Denture appearance, fit, and odor; also concerns about how to manage them during intimate moments
- Changes in body fat distribution
- Loss of vigor and strength
- Inability to exercise and to ambulate independently (including embarrassment over the use of a walker or wheelchair)

It is notable that many of the body image-related concerns espoused by elderly women do not focus on appearance per se, but on sensory deficits and changes in body function (e.g., incontinence and arthritic stiffness) that impair a woman's autonomy. Because many sensory deficits make it more difficult for elderly women to groom and dress themselves, many of these women cite additional concerns that their loss of independence makes them feel less vigorous and sensual. For others, a loss in hearing, vision, or taste means that they are not able to gain as much enjoyment from previously enjoyable sensual activities such as listening to classical music, admiring beautiful art, or savoring a gourmet meal.

Practical Issues

To complicate practical matters further, the fashion industry has not yet met increasing demands for elderly women and their sometimes special needs for clothing (Chrisler & Ghiz, 1993; Jackson & O'Neal, 1982). Elderly women who have arthritis or other ailments that result in difficulties with manual dexterity may need clothing with large fasteners, buttons, or Velcro patches to allow them to dress independently. A large dowager's hump may make it difficult to find blouses or dresses that have enough fullness through the upper back to fit properly and comfortably. Because of certain medical conditions and poor circulation, some older women must find clothing that provides additional warmth indoors as well as comfort and good looks. Only a few specialty stores and catalogue houses offer such clothing, as the clothing industry has yet to recognize this growing market in the population (Jackson & O'Neal, 1982). In response, many elderly women either stop shopping altogether or are forced to buy extralarge sizes and perhaps have them altered. Others lament that while shopping used to be an enjoyable, sociable activity that allowed them to affirm their femininity, it has evolved into an unpleasant chore that serves as an unpleasant reminder of their bodies' undesirable changes in appearance and function.

## EATING DISORDERS

A dangerous assumption made by some health care providers is that eating disorders are manifested primarily among adolescent and young adult women. In the past 30 years, the numbers of patients diagnosed with eating disorders including bulimia and anorexia nervosa have increased dramatically. Because some proportion of these women (perhaps as many as 20%) tend to develop chronic symptoms (Hsu, Crisp, & Harding, 1979; Theander, 1985), one would expect that these younger women develop into older women with eating disorders (Hsu & Zimmer, 1988). Although the specific etiology for eating disorders is unknown, women with a history of comorbid depression or personality disorder may be at greater risk for maintaining these disorders into late life (Hsu & Zimmer, 1988).

What may be more insidious about the prevalence of eating disorders in late life is that within the past few years, there have been documented cases in the literature of older women developing eating disorders for the *first* time in old age (e.g., Hsu & Zimmer, 1988; Jonas, Pope, Hudson, & Satlin, 1984; Price, Gianni, & Colella, 1985). The increasingly intense pressure on women from all age groups to maintain a youthful, slim appearance can be expected to contribute to this emergence of symptoms in later life (Hsu & Zimmer, 1988). An empirical study of more than 100 elderly women revealed that the women in the sample believed that weight loss was directly correlated with "youthful looks" (Gupta & Schork, 1993). Given this internalization of societal demands for youth and thinness, clinicians can expect to see more elderly female (and male; Ronch, 1985) patients presenting with eating disorders and disturbances in body image.

Clinicians should be particularly alert to any elderly patient who is described as a "problem eater" by staff members in an institutional setting (Ronch, 1985), or to any rapid fluctuations or change in weight among community-living patients. Most importantly, one must be careful not to assume that rapid weight loss among an older female patient represents a stressful response to aging or a response to a chronic illness. An interdisciplinary team approach that includes therapists, geriatricians, and nutritionists, coupled with a thorough intake interview about binging, purging, and body image, can help reveal a more complete diagnostic picture.

Ruth

Ruth was a 68-year-old divorced woman who moved to a nursing home because her rheumatoid arthritis and advanced glaucoma prevented her from caring for herself independently. She used a walker to ambulate, and was not able to drive because of her diminished vision. Instead of moving in with relatives, Ruth decided to move into a nursing home. She had no children, and only a tense relationship with a niece who lived in the area. While at the nursing home, Ruth presented with depression and symptoms of an eating disorder. She would eat her meals in the dining room, but would often pick at her food and rearrange it on the plate rather than eat it. One nursing assistant observed Ruth placing spoonfuls of vegetables and meat into an empty milk container, ostensibly to make it look as though she had eaten more of her meal. It also was unclear whether Ruth purged by vomiting after meals. She had a private bathroom in her room, and staff members were unclear as to how closely they should (or could, for ethical reasons) monitor her. When asked by staff members why she was not eating or if she was making herself vomit after she did eat, Ruth responded with a flat denial. However, she was overheard to tell other patients that she was on a diet because she was "so big and fat." In reality, Ruth was within the normal weight for a woman her size and age.

After one outing with her niece, Ruth returned to the nursing home in tears. When approached by the staff psychologist, Ruth admitted that she was so upset because her niece always rushed her when they were shopping. When asked about it further, Ruth described how frustrated she was about her inability to find pants that fit over her thighs and her dowager's hump. "I can't stand it!... Everything just fits wrong and I look so big and fat and ugly!... And, she just rushes and rushes me ... she doesn't care, but I do.... I can't stand it." Ruth then admitted that she was trying to diet because she felt that if she lost enough weight, she might be able to fit into some of her older clothes that she liked, and not have to go shopping anymore. When pressed, she said that she believed if she lost enough weight, her thighs would shrink and her dowager's hump might even get smaller, despite her physician's information to the contrary. She also admitted to starving herself at times, and using her finger to make herself vomit in the bathroom after she ate a dessert or a "starchy food" like pasta or a baked potato. Because of the professional concern and willingness of the staff members to put aside age-related stereotypes that eating disorders were exhibited exclusively among younger adults, Ruth was interviewed and diagnosed with bulimia. With the support of the staff psychologist, she agreed to begin a program of treatment.

## EXACERBATION OF EXISTING CLINICAL PATHOLOGY

Women with longstanding psychological disorders also are at increased risk for body image disturbances. Depression and psychotic depression certainly foster inaccurate perceptions of a changing, aging body. Because psychotic depression is often undiagnosed among elderly adults, as it often is assumed to be a symptom of dementia, many elderly women may develop delusions about their appearance or body function. For elderly women with narcissistic or histrionic personality disorder, aging itself poses many egregious developmental tasks. For a woman who has narcissistic traits, the use of a cane for increasingly severe arthritis can be viewed as an assault against the self. Even being around other older adults who are naturally showing signs of their age can be taken as a narcissistic assault as the personality-disordered older woman is literally forced to see what does not mirror her own needs and expectations. An older woman with histrionic traits who may have relied heavily on her abilities to relate to members of the opposite sex in primarily sexualized ways may feel at a loss if she perceives that her "looks are gone," and her prior means of attracting attention are not as effective. With him, she will need to learn to depend on more adaptive, collaborative modes of interaction to establish relationships with and gain attention from others.

Fortunately, both dynamic and cognitive–behavioral approaches in therapy can be employed effectively in order to assist elderly women in coping with some of the bodily changes that they experience with age. From the dynamic perspective, an exploration of internalized object relations can help older women acknowledge that a previous sense of self that was based primarily on outward, physical characteristics is bound to suffer with age. Allowing elderly women to acknowledge, accept, and grieve their perceptions of lost youth and independence will allow for more adaptive coping behaviors to emerge. A more global, integrated view of the self will emerge that will allow elderly women to view their aging bodies as "outward signs of inner wisdom" (Chrisler & Ghiz, 1993). Cognitive–behavioral measures also are helpful in fostering adaptive coping with physical aging. Techniques such as occupational therapy, dance therapy (Unger, 1985), and structured exercise programs have been shown to increase elderly women's self-esteem and improve their body image (O'Brien & Vertinsky, 1990). Even though an older woman may have limited strength and mobility, exercising or dancing to music while sitting in a chair or in a bed from a prone position can generate significant benefits.

### Yolonda

Yolonda was a 71-year-old woman who attended a partial day hospitalization program for depression. She had never married, had been a successful stenographer, and had maintained her own apartment for the last 45 years. During the past year, however, Yolonda began to develop glaucoma. She had always enjoyed needlepoint, and said that she became depressed when she could no longer pursue her hobby and when she had difficulty crossing the street and shopping by herself. It had become almost impossible for her to see oncoming cars or to read the prices on items in the store. She was admitted to the day hospital program when the woman who helped her with meals and laundry each day noticed that Yolonda was no longer eating and that she would not get out of bed.

After being in the program for a few weeks, Yolonda began to make friendships with some of the other women. She began to explore knitting and listening to music as other possible hobbies. (She could "feel" the needles and stitches for knitting.) As the therapeutic relationship grew between Yolonda and her therapist, Yolonda began to address other issues that lent themselves to her depression. She noted that she had been in love with a young man in her early 20s, but that he had died tragically in a car accident. She had other offers for dating and even for marriage, but Yolonda felt that she could only have loved this one man. Now that she was approaching the last decade of her life, however, she sometimes regretted her decision not to seek a companion.

When asked how she felt about trying to date or find a companion at this point in her life, she responded flatly, "How can I with this hair?" Her therapist was curious, as Yolonda was an attractive older woman with shoulder-length gray hair. She inquired as to what was wrong with her hair, and Yolonda acted very surprised. She expressed concern that her therapist couldn't understand that with "no hair," no one would possibly think she was attractive. In fact, Yolonda literally meant that she had no hair; she had a circumscribed delusion that her hair had been falling out in clumps, and that she was almost bald. She said that she tried to always "dress nice," and sometimes even wear makeup, but that she was too anxious about her hair to even think about dating. When her therapist attempted to explore the delusion carefully, and asked what Yolonda saw in the mirror or when she brushed her hair, Yolonda simply shrugged and said, "I suppose sometimes it is worse than others.... I guess a part of me does think I have hair ... but that doesn't last for very long."

After intensive therapy in which Yolonda explored her ambivalence about closeness and intimacy with men, her major depression began to subside. Through work with an interdisciplinary team, Yolonda also received some psychotropic medication to help alleviate her psychotic depression. After another few weeks, Yolonda's ego strength became strengthened. She was able to recognize that she did, in fact, have thick hair, but that it was her fears about becoming close to others that allowed her to think that she had no hair. Yolonda's therapist also was accepting and patient in that Yolonda's delusions were very real to her, and that they must be taken seriously. Ultimately, this elderly woman recognized that she did not have to have male companionship to feel loved and attractive. With intensive therapy and medication management, she was able to develop caring friendships, mourn the loss of her eyesight, and adopt more suitable hobbies. Although it remained unclear whether Yolonda had never resolved or mourned the loss of her first love or whether she had an unexplored homosexual orientation, this elderly woman ultimately was able to discount her body image distortion and feel pride and acceptance in her appearance. Her distortions in body image were taken seriously, and were thus treated appropriately by all members of the treatment team.

## Nancy

Nancy was an 89-year-old woman who resided in a nursing home. She was known by staff members as one of the most challenging patients in the facility. Nancy had been diagnosed with narcissistic personality disorder, and often made inappropriate demands on both staff members and other patients. Throughout her life, Nancy had relied on sexuality and her appearance for her sense of self-esteem, approval, and womanhood. Quite simply, because of poor internal object relations developed ostensibly through poor modeling by her parents and significant others at a young age, Nancy literally sought out others to mirror and appreciate her own external image. Her only sense of self was what she saw reflected in the eyes of others. In the nursing home, Nancy consistently demanded that others acknowledge her presence, and even would go so far as to say that she would only wear pink, blue, and purple as they were "the colors of royalty and princesses." Nancy also would only associate with other residents who were at least as healthy as her. She said that she could not tolerate "having to look at old, sick people," and sometimes would refuse to eat in the dining room if certain patients in wheelchairs were present.

Although she was sometimes a management problem, staff members could often effectively use limit setting and behavioral (i.e., token economy) techniques with her. However, Nancy's behavior soon escalated after she fell in the bathroom and broke her hip, requiring immediate surgery for a hip replacement. After the surgery, Nancy was forced to rely on a wheelchair to ambulate, and was told that she needed to attend physical therapy daily in order to guarantee the success of the procedure. The staff psychologist was asked to see Nancy after she had began to refuse her physical therapy treatments, and her physician, physical therapist, and occupational therapist could not persuade her to continue.

During therapy, Nancy's therapist recognized that making any long term personality changes was highly unlikely in the short term, and she focused instead on encouraging Nancy to articulate her feelings in order to encourage her to attend her physical therapy sessions. Nancy became a regular participant in twice-weekly psychotherapy, and began to tell her therapist about her desires to be wealthy, independent, and beautiful. "You know, I was quite a woman in my day.... I turned heads.... I wore all the right clothes in the right way, if you know what I mean." When asked gently how she felt now that she was older, and had an unfortunate fall, Nancy was able to vent her anger and articulate some of her narcissistic injuries, "This is a disgrace.... I can't even get myself to the bathroom ... what's the point now, anyway?" Once she vented some of her anger and frustration (most of the staff members were so frustrated with Nancy that it was difficult for them to tolerate, much less entertain her constant tirades and complaints), Nancy was willing to go to some of her appointments. However, the physical therapists and nursing aides often spent more than 30 minutes yelling, screaming, talking, and begging in order for her to attend. The situation was spiraling out of control, and Nancy's narcissistic needs were being met in an interpersonally maladaptive way. She was gaining significant attention, but only because she was being passive, argumentative, and demanding.

Nancy's therapist then educated the nursing home staff members about the fear underlying Nancy's refusal to attend physical therapy. (Confidentiality issues were not broached in any of these discussions.) With guidance, the physical therapists were willing to set limits for Nancy, and to only give her positive reinforcement when she did attend her sessions. For example, staff members were instructed to ask Nancy to attend her session once in the morning, and to give her only one reminder a few minutes before her appointment. They also were told not to cajole or beg Nancy to attend her appointment, but to stress to her that it was her personal choice and responsibility to attend therapy; they would respect *her* wishes. This tactic provided Nancy with some sense of dignity and control, and forced her to move from a passive-dependent position to a more assertive one in which she gained attention and mirroring by engaging in adaptive behaviors. The physical therapists also provided a spontaneous therapeutic intervention for Nancy in which they crafted a homemade birthday card for her that included the phrases "sexy lady," "beautiful," and "fun and feisty."

Through the combination of appropriate direction and support from her therapist, physical therapists, and other support staff, Nancy soon regained her mobility. In the short run, her personality structure became less rigid, and a more behavioral approach allowed her to complete her sometimes painful trial of physical therapy. Nancy also went on in therapy to work on changing some established patterns in her interpersonal relationships, and was able to develop more positive coping skills in response to her changing body image.

## UNEXPECTED POSITIVE CHANGES

Although the majority of elderly women report some level of discomfort or disdain regarding their body image, some elderly women maintain positive attitudes toward their bodies and appearance throughout life. In fact, others actually grow to enjoy a level of comfort with their body for the first time in late life. It thus is important that practitioners ask their elderly female patients about their body image, rather than simply assume that their emerging perceptions to be negative and disturbing.

### Amy

One elderly woman reported that she had been considered very beautiful when she was younger; everywhere she went she heard cat calls, whistles, and shouts. Amy described that she was constantly approached by a variety of men, whether she was out shopping at the grocery store or at a nightclub with a date. She found it sometimes difficult to make female friends; they often felt jealous and threatened by her appearance. Some female acquaintances even told her that they wouldn't introduce her to their husbands. What upset Amy even more was that she felt that no one ever took her seriously. "After all," she said, "back then, beautiful women were automatically assumed to be dimwitted ... maybe they thought you could be a model or a dancer ... people didn't even think I could possibly be a good secretary ... no one would even ask me who I voted for in the elections."

Once Amy reached her mid-50s and 60s, however, she found that it was a huge relief to walk on the street without being "a target" any more. She described having a refreshing sense of freedom to go where she wanted, when she wanted without living in fear or notoriety. Amy also found it was easier to begin friendships with women, and that both men and women seemed to be more interested in what she had to say than what she looked like. Near the completion of her therapy, Amy enrolled in a college course in politics at the local community college and felt validated by her scholastic performance. Her therapist allowed Amy to recognize both the positive and negative aspects in her assumption of the role as "blond bombshell," and how she may have played a part in perpetuating this dynamic in the form of a self-fulfilling prophesy. But for now, age had leveled the playing field for Amy, and it allowed both herself and others to focus on her inner qualities instead of exclusively on her outward appearance.

## BREAST AND CERVICAL CANCER

In any responsible discussion of female sexuality, the detection and treatment of breast and cervical cancer must be addressed. This aspect of female sexuality has become particularly salient among the growing population of older adult women. As women age, their risk for both breast cancer and cervical cancer increases (e.g., Eddy, 1989; Greenwald & Sondik, 1986). Despite this age-related increase in pathology, epidemiological studies show consistently that older women, compared to their younger counterparts, are also significantly less likely to have mammograms (Rimer, Ross, Cristinzio, & King, 1992) or pap smears on a regular basis (Ives, Lave, Traven, Schultz, & Kuller, 1996; Marwill, Freund, & Barry, 1996), despite their greater use of primary health care services (Love, Davis, Mundt, & Clark, 1997).

### Detection

Women who are least likely to be screened for breast and cervical cancers include those who live in rural areas, who are from a low socioeconomic status, depressed (Ives et al., 1996), single or divorced (Makuc, Freid, & Kleinman, 1989), and without an HMO insurance plan (Love et al., 1997). Among minority group members, including Hispanic elders, researchers also have identified embarrassment (Morisky, Fox, Murata, & Stein, 1989) as a barrier for screening. Some researchers suggest that an internalized stereotype that age is equated

with illness, coupled with a lack of overall social support, contributes significantly to elderly women's poor participation in cancer screening (Pizzi & Wolf,
1998). In support of this supposition, surveys of more than 3000 elderly women
from urban and rural areas showed that the majority were unaware of their need
for breast cancer screening (Ives et al., 1996), and that many felt that mammograms were necessary only if they already showed symptoms of cancer such as
discharge or bleeding (Rimer et al., 1992).

Although little is known about elderly women's knowledge of cervical
cancer, studies suggest that many of them are not aware that pap smears detect
the presence of cervical cancer in its early stages and that the virus responsible is
transmitted through sexual contact (Ives et al., 1996). Although the American
Cancer Society suggests that if three consecutive, annual pap smears have
revealed a negative result, pelvic exams and pap smears need only be conducted
every 3 years for elderly adults, physicians may not even ask an elderly women
if she is sexually active and acknowledge the need for more frequent testing.
Compounding the problem further, physicians themselves have been shown to
profess only partial agreement with the American Cancer Society's guidelines
for annual mammography for elderly women (e.g., American Cancer Society,
1985; Dietrich et al., 1992), and have shown less interest in recommending
mammograms for oldest-old women (aged 75 and older), for women with dementia, and for women living in nursing homes (Marwill, Freund, & Barry,
1996). Fortunately, elderly women who have been educated about cancer risks
and who have been invited to participate in screening programs have shown
similar rates of compliance as their younger counterparts (Taylor, McPherson,
Parbhoo, & Perry, 1996).

Treatment

In addition to difficulties in obtaining appropriate physician referrals, patient interest, and compliance with cancer screening measures (e.g., Fletcher,
Morgan, O'Malley, Earp, & Degnan, 1989), treatment issues regarding breast and
cervical cancer among elderly women typically pose significant medical, ethical, and psychological problems. Although a psychotherapist certainly is not
qualified to make medical diagnoses and treatment plans regarding breast
lumps, abnormal pap smears, and breast and cervical cancers, primary therapists can assist their patients in coping emotionally with their individual barriers to screening, and with their potentially abnormal test results. Many elderly
women are intimidated by their physicians, particularly if their physicians
themselves are not comfortable discussing issues of sexuality with their patients. Psychologists and other mental health care practitioners also may be
able to assist family members in identifying and articulating their views about
screening and treatment for an elderly mother or aunt who may be unable to
make appropriate decisions for herself because of dementia or other chronic
mental illness.

Questions also may be raised about whether treatment for breast or cervical
cancer will provide an increase in quality of life for an elderly woman, or

whether these treatments will only induce pain and suffering that exceeds any benefits in decreased mortality. A variety of survival benefit curves and predictions based on general population statistics are available to assist patients and physicians in determining treatment course (e.g., Robinson & Balducci, 1995). However, care must be taken to incorporate quality of life issues (e.g., pain relief and the ability of family members to provide care outside of an institutional setting) and religious preferences into any otherwise sterile discussion. Such tasks can be made even more difficult if an elderly patient diagnosed with cancer is impaired mentally. For example, is it appropriate to order a mastectomy without obtaining the older woman's permission? For older women who are quite capable of making their own decisions about whether to undergo a mastectomy in the face of breast cancer, for example, some concerns may be raised that medical personnel can significantly underestimate the elderly woman's duress on undergoing disfiguring, major surgery. Some health care providers may feel that for an older woman, particularly for one who is widowed or single, breast loss is not as emotionally difficult or as central to their identity as it would be for younger women. For a number of older women, many feel that their breast represents one of their only remaining, concrete reminders of their femininity in the face of chronic illness and age. It becomes vital to provide open lines of inquiry regarding invasive medical procedures that may alter a woman's physical appearance. On discussion, some physicians are able to consider reconstructive surgery after mastectomy if their patients request it.

In sum, what is most important for mental health providers is to assist their patients in communicating effectively with their physicians, caregivers, friends, and family members in order to provide the most effective treatment plan. Empirical research suggests that older women would benefit from an advocate and supporter during treatment planning; older women with breast cancer have been shown to seek less information about their treatment options and make hastier decisions about their treatment than younger women (Meyer, Russo, & Talbot, 1995). It also is important to recognize and respect the fact that for some elderly women, aggressive treatment for breast or cervical cancer is their preferred choice, whereas the withholding of treatment becomes the preferred choice for others. As effective clinicians, we must inform and support our older female patients in their difficult decision making, without imposing our own moral and religious views.

## SUMMARY

Older women are faced with conflicting messages from society about their role as women, sexual beings, and potential contributors to society. These societal demands placed on elderly women, coupled with their own internalized stereotypes and expectations, can be enormous, and may be inappropriately internalized and manifested in the form of sexual dysfunction or dissatisfaction, body image distortions, depression, eating disorders, or poor participation in breast and cervical cancer screenings among others. Because of a general lack of knowledge among the health care community as well as the general population, most elderly women are not aware of the *normal*, basic physiological changes that take place with age, stemming primarily from a decrease in production of estrogen. Many older women are delighted to learn that treatments are available to assist them in coping with changes in their sexual response cycle, in order to restore their enjoyment in sexual activity. Clinicians also need to acknowledge the sensual as well as sexual needs of elderly female patients, who may be with or without a partner. There is no reason why an elderly woman cannot enjoy and relish her status as a woman throughout the life span.

# 8

# Men's Issues in Elderly Sexuality

*In nearly all cultures, the functioning of the male phallus is tied intimately to a man's sense of self, body image, and implied social worth. Although empirical studies suggest consistently that elderly men engage in sexual activity into late life with a relatively high frequency, more anecdotal, clinical evidence suggests that older men may regard age-related changes in their sexual response cycle with trepidation, embarrassment, anger, and fear.*

## HISTORICAL AND SOCIETAL VALUES

One of the cornerstones of Freud's theory was his articulation of the differences between male and female sexuality and sexuality's overall relation to personality functioning and development. The penis, as reflected in its importance as an external sexual organ (as compared to the internalized, female uterus), was paramount. From early childhood, women were thought to envy the penis both symbolically and literally. The penis represented something that a woman was "missing" as well as more general opportunities to advance and enact change in a male-dominated society. Although it can be argued that Freud was a champion of women in that he took their views seriously, promoted nonsexualized physician–patient relationships, and believed that psychic trauma, and not an inflamed uterus, for example, could be responsible for neuroses and psychosomatic symptoms, he was steeped in his culture and championed the inherent position and power of men. The psychological price to be paid for such an emphasis on male anatomy is that men could be expected to experience castration anxiety in the presence of aggressive women and mothers, competing fathers, and personal failures at home or at work.

Popular culture reflects this general emphasis on the male sexual organ and its imbued abilities to wield power and foster competition. Consider the pervasive use of slang and curse words to illustrate the power of the penis: fuck you; bite me; you suck; eat me; stick it; this blows; piss off; dick head; jerk off; and he's got balls. There are no such parallel expressions regarding female anatomy. Something is inexorably tied between the penis and competition, aggression, and physical satisfaction in the public eye. Media moguls know that older men such as Clint Eastwood, Warren Beatty, and Sean Connery can still command large audiences as action heroes and sex symbols. It is much more common and socially acceptable for older men to marry and date younger women. For better or worse, sex and power are intertwined in our culture, particularly in the male venue. As a corollary, any sexual dysfunction among men (caused by physiological or psychological difficulties) must be taken seriously as a significant psychological assault.

## PHYSIOLOGICAL CHANGES

Even though aging is certainly not a pathological process, normal aging typically produces some changes in male sexual functioning. Most elderly male patients are unfamiliar with these changes, and may become frightened or confused when they experience them. A mental health practitioner can serve as a conduit between an elderly male patient and a sensitive and informed urologist, internist, or geriatrician when it appears that physiological problems may underlie such sexual changes. Sometimes the dissemination of knowledge of these age-related changes is enough to ease the mind of older male patients and to encourage them to take proactive measures and resume their enjoyment of sexual activity.

Sexual Response Cycle

There is substantial debate about whether men experience age-related hormonal changes as women do in menopause (e.g., Morley, 1996). These hormonally related changes have been referred to as viropause or manopause, and are believed to be associated with a very gradual decline in the production of testicular testosterone in men sometime after the age of 50. More specifically, some researchers attribute a general loss in sexual interest (i.e., loss of libido) and a decrease in the ability to obtain and maintain an erection (i.e., loss of potency) to this decline in androgen production (Kaiser & Morley, 1994; Morley, 1996; Schiavi et al., 1991). Alternatively, other researchers maintain that testosterone production has little to do with an ability to maintain an erection (Segraves & Segraves, 1995); vascular disease appears to play a major role (Kaiser et al., 1988). Regardless of the role of testosterone in the maintenance of normal sexual function, debate continues to ensue about the reality of such a developmentally based hormonal decline among men.

Whether or not a specific event is responsible for changes in the sexual response cycle among older men, a number of age-related changes are typically observed (e.g., Galindo & Kaiser, 1995; Meston, 1997; Schiavi & Rehman, 1995):

- Loss of sexual desire or libido
- Decrease in vasocongestion (blood flow) to the scrotum
- Reduced tension in the scrotal sac both before and during intercourse
- Delay in time required to achieve erection

- Decrease in penile sensitivity
- Increase in time required for orgasm and ejaculation
- Gradual decline in overall amount of semen expelled at orgasm

Some older men find that while they were once able to achieve an erection in seconds, they may now require a few minutes to achieve arousal sufficient for penetration. This may not necessarily indicate underlying pathology; a decrease in the number of adrenergic and cholinergic receptors may interfere with smooth muscle relaxation and the rapid, autonomic flow of blood to the penis to produce an erection (e.g., Schiavi & Rehman, 1995). Panic is common for older men who are unaware that this time delay in achieving erection is normal in many regards. Many older men immediately jump to the conclusion that they are impotent and quite unnecessarily cease involvement in sexual activity.

Because older men also may experience a general decline in sexual desire, their partners may or may not question whether their attractiveness or desirability is in decline. Other partners and spouses may become confused, frustrated, or angry when they find that they are asked, or simply need, to physically stimulate their partner's penis in order for him to achieve arousal. One long-time spouse remarked, "I always thought it was just good enough for him to just see me naked.... Now he wants me to touch him with my hands and my mouth.... We haven't done that sort of thing in many years.... Why aren't I good enough the way I am?... Is this some sick fantasy of his or is he having an affair and maybe *she* does those things?" Communication between partners can become critical. It also is typical (but not an appropriate assumption) for a female partner to place less emphasis on the actual quality of her spouse's erection than on the quality of their foreplay or on their relationship in general. Many older men are distressed deeply that they "can't get things going" as quickly as they used to, and feel powerless and embarrassed. Learning that their partner is willing to discuss the issue and even downplay it in some instances can alleviate further performance anxiety in elderly men.

Not all age-related changes in the male sexual response cycle are inherently negative. For example, elderly men who previously experienced difficulties with premature ejaculation, an increased need for physical stimulation, and a slower buildup to orgasm can prolong the sexual act, which can be associated with greater enjoyment for both partners. Some older men have described feeling free to enjoy themselves and their sexual partners now that they no longer have to worry about "holding back" or "controlling themselves" during intercourse. Other women have reported that they enjoy the slower pace of their love making now that their husband "takes his time" and seems to enjoy himself instead of rushing to climax. Again, open communication and basic education among both partners (often assisted by a clinician) can be critical.

Assessment

Proper interviewing and assessment is vital to assisting older men in discussing previously undisclosed issues in order to foster patient education, interpersonal exploration, and consultations with appropriate medical specialists when necessary. Open-ended questions and questions that assume the presence of some difficulties may make it easier for initially reluctant patients to respond. Sometimes the presence of a younger, female clinician can be cause for concern among older male patients who may not be accustomed to women as professionals or who were raised in a cohort in which it was considered inappropriate to discuss sexual matters with women. If a patient appears reluctant to discuss sexual concerns with a female professional, a frank discussion of the patient's concerns is in order. Similar issues can arise when an older male patient is confronted with a younger male clinician. Most patients respond very positively when their clinician is willing to address the "process" as well as the "content" of their interview. Sometimes simply asking, "What is it like for me to ask you these questions about sex?... Some people do find it a little unsettling at first" is enough to engender a meaningful discussion of the patient's underlying anxieties, fears, and social mores. Once these issues are addressed, a more open discussion of a patient's sexual concerns and symptoms is likely to follow.

A number of standard questions can be addressed during a patient interview, or when a patient in longer term therapy suddenly announces concerns about sexual function. These include (e.g., Galindo & Kaiser, 1995; Sbrocco, Weisberg, & Barlow, 1995):

- Most people have some difficulties with sex at some point in their lives. What concerns do you have about your sex life or sexual functioning?
- How do you think your partner feels about your sex life?
- What do you think constitutes a satisfying sex life? How would you compare your own sex life to your idea of a satisfying or "perfect" sex life?
- How often do you masturbate? Do you ever have any trouble masturbating? What kind of trouble do you have?
- Are your sexual partners, both now or previously, primarily women or men? Have you ever had any same-sex sexual encounters? Have you ever had sex with a prostitute? With an intravenous drug user? (Be *sure* to consider the patient's religious beliefs carefully when asking such questions regarding high risk behaviors and masturbation.)
- How do you feel about your body? Are you happy with it or are there some things that worry you, or that you wish could be different? Have you ever tried to change anything about your body? How are your eating habits?
- How difficult is it for you to talk about sex with your partner? Have you ever talked about anything in particular?
- How difficult is it to get a full erection during sex? During masturbation?
- How often do you get erections? Are they as firm as you would like them to be, or as they used to be?
- Is it ever painful when having sex?
- Are you able to orgasm/come/ejaculate?
- How interested or disinterested are you in sex? Is this level of interest different than before?

- Do you ever have trouble or pain when urinating? Do you need to go to the bathroom more often than you would like? Has your prostate ever been checked?
- What medical problems do you have? What have you been diagnosed with?
- What prescription medications are you currently taking? What over-the-counter medications do you take, even on an occasional basis?
- How often do you smoke, drink alcohol, or use drugs?

Note that issues involving masturbation, quality of communication between partners, participation in high risk behaviors, underlying medical conditions, concerns about one's overall appearance, and overall interest in sex are just as important as specific questions about the presence and firmness of an erection. Older male patients often benefit from this implicit message that their global sense of sexuality and self is at least as important as the singular functioning of their penis.

## BODY IMAGE AND RELATED PROBLEMS

Because women are traditionally viewed as sex objects who are supposed to remain thin, beautiful, and youthful in order to gain companionship and vital resources, men's concerns about body image, body functioning, and overall appearance are often overlooked as minimal or unimportant. One commonly overlooked problem among older men is that of distortions in body image. Some of these more distressing age-related changes for men are likely to include an overall decline in physical strength and stamina, male pattern baldness, and gynecomastia (enlargement of the fatty tissue of the breast).

Empirical studies have suggested that although men view their bodies in a variety of ways, they often focus on three primary aspects of their body: upper body strength, physical stamina, and level of attractiveness (Brown, Cash, & Mikulka, 1990; Franzoi & Shields, 1984). The few empirical studies that exist regarding older men's body image suggest that throughout midlife and old age, men appear to place significantly less emphasis on their body image than women (Cash, Winstead, & Janda, 1986; Plutchik, Conte, & Weiner, 1973; Plutchik, Weiner, & Conte, 1971). Consistent with these findings, the vast majority of young and older people suffering from eating disorders are women. However, a small percentage of those afflicted are men, who are equally deserving of clinicians' and researchers' time and attention (e.g., Van Deusen, 1997). Like their female counterparts, men with anorexia and bulimia tend to choose an inappropriate ideal for their body image which is too thin for their normal height and body frame (Barry & Lippmann, 1990). Many times older male patients who lose a significant amount of weight in a short period of time are assumed to be just depressed or "[physically] sick." Stereotypes persist that elderly adults simply lose interest in food and other activities as they age. It becomes vital for informed clinicians to assess for the presence of distortions in body image or a related eating disorder whenever conducting an initial interview.

Another common concern among older men is that of baldness (e.g., Morley, 1996). Male pattern baldness has generated a multimillion dollar industry that boasts realistic and unrealistic claims for treatment including toupees, hair transplants, and drug therapies. The fact that this is a multimillion dollar industry highlights the psychological difficulties that many middle-aged and older men endure as they experience hair loss. One 76-year-old man commented, "Well, I can cover up the rest of me with nice suits and shirts and things, but I can't do too much with this chrome dome.... I don't like wearing a hat inside, and besides, I'm afraid that wearing a hat will make me lose even more [hair] ... my wife doesn't seem to mind, but it does get to me every now and then." It also remains unclear why some older men adjust well to hair loss whereas others do not. Some men indicate that baldness is a problem because it makes them unattractive to women, whereas others point out that every time they look in the mirror, they are given a painful reminder of their aging bodies, even if they had been feeling good about themselves the moment before they glanced in the mirror. On a practical level, other older men cite concerns about sunburn and skin cancer on their exposed scalp. More psychoanalytic approaches view preoccupation with hair as a narcissistic defense against the uncovering of some aspect of the self. This view is consistent with the general assumption that hair loss in men presents itself as an undeniable reminder of aging.

A significantly less discussed but equally problematic age-related change for some older men is that of gynecomastia (Morley, 1996). The majority of men experience either a subtle or dramatic change in the fatty composition of their chest, specifically in their breasts (Carlson, 1980). This increase in fatty tissue may first present itself in one breast only, and may require a visit to a physician to rule out breast cancer. Traditionally, this increase in fatty tissue takes place in both breasts and is, for better or worse, a sign of normal aging. The only available medical treatment is breast reduction surgery; hormonal treatments do not appear to be safe or effective (Carlson, 1980). Some older men simply respond to this body change by noting, "Well, it's about time for me to get old and flabby, I guess." Others attempt to hide their chests by wearing large shirts or suits with heavily padded shoulders. One 83-year-old man articulated his distress by stating, "I mean, I look like a girl ... it's embarrassing just to take my shirt off. I don't even know the last time I went swimming." Sometimes educating the patient about the normality of this event is enough to allow him to feel more comfortable with his body's changes. At other times, a discussion of these issues leads to important therapeutic work in differentiating male and female roles, identifying distortions in body imagery, and uncovering homophobic or homosexual tendencies.

## IMPOTENCE

Impotence, the inability to achieve erection or to achieve an erection that is firm enough for masturbation or penetration, is one of the most feared symptoms of sexual dysfunction among men. It also is the most common source of sexual dysfunction among older men (National Institutes of Health, 1993). Many older men are reluctant to even discuss the issue, and are not likely to be cognizant of the underlying medical problems, surgical procedures, and side effects from prescription medications that can cause impotence. To compound the problem further, many clinicians employ stereotypes that older men do not have a need for vaginal intercourse anyway, and that it simply becomes a matter of helping these men enjoy "other" sexual activities (Butler et al., 1994). In contrast, studies suggest that men from certain socioeconomic groups actually cease participation in all heterosexual activity if they become impotent and unable to achieve penetration with their partner (Cogen & Steinman, 1990). In other cases, a clinician's cultural or religious background inhibits a discussion of the importance of the patient's problem. It thus becomes the clinician's first responsibility to help an older male patient discover the underlying cause of his impotence and to look for both medical and psychological means to ameliorate the problem. Only as an absolute last resort should an older man be told, in effect, "Well, this is a significant loss that will have to be recognized, discussed, and mourned.... We can work together to help you discover other types of things you can do to get some sexual pleasure."

## Mike

Mike was a 66-year-old single man who was admitted to a psychiatric facility on court order following a suicide attempt. He had been scheduled to go through a painful rectal procedure and took a bottle of sleeping pills the night before in order to avoid going through the surgery. At the time, he had been unemployed and homeless for the last 6 months and was staying with his financially successful older sister and her husband. Mike engaged reluctantly in psychotherapy, primarily because he acknowledged that if he were not willing to discuss his suicide attempt he was not likely to be released from the unit any time soon. He was diagnosed with major depression and dependent personality disorder. On the unit he was passive aggressive and had difficulty discussing his own needs and wants. Mike began to progress in therapy, and recognized that his yelling outbursts ostracized him from the family members he cared most about, and that he could find more assertive ways to deal with his problems. He began to explore his feelings of failure as a younger man and acknowledge that his suicide attempt was a way to gain attention from his family members, to make his family members feel guilty, and to avoid taking responsibility for his own health. He also agreed to take antidepressant medication at the request of the staff psychiatrist.

Three weeks into treatment, Mike discussed his difficulties in finding a "steady girlfriend." His suicide attempt was preceded by his previous girlfriend's abrupt termination of a yearlong relationship after he lost his job as a masonry worker because of layoffs. He expressed a desire to be married, but feared that he was getting too old for anybody to want him, particularly with his sporadic work history and moderate level of income. He also told his therapist that he was having trouble with some things "down there, you know?" When his therapist said that she wanted to understand what he meant by that, Mike said that he "had trouble, you know, moving things along, getting things into place, when [he was] out on a date with a woman." He said that he didn't even want to go on dates when he knew that if "things started getting close ... I couldn't deliver." His therapist assured him that these were very important concerns, and suggested that while they discuss the possible impact of his recent breakup with his last girlfriend on his ability to "be prepared," he simultaneously ask the staff psychiatrist about possible, underlying medical causes for his problem. (Only the staff psychiatrist could make other medical referrals.) The therapist also approached Mike's psychiatrist privately and informed her that he was gathering the courage to schedule an appointment with her to discuss a particularly sensitive issue.

A few sessions later, Mike seemed particularly angry and morose. When his therapist asked him if something triggered his abrupt change in mood, he answered bitterly, "That bitch said that it wasn't something I should be worried about—that I have more important things to work on like not being so depressed.... What the hell does she know? Maybe I'm depressed because I can't get it up, you know?... She said that she might make a referral for me to see a urologist in 'a month or so if it's still bothering [me].' You know, what the fuck is that?" The therapist quickly mirrored Mike's frustration with his inability to get important information, and more importantly, his inability to be taken seriously. (The therapist also had to work carefully to avoid making a split in the treatment team by offering unprofessional comments regarding the staff psychiatrist.) Mike's initial response to his psychiatrist's snafu was to have his therapist approach her instead and "do it for me, would you?... You obviously know her better than I do, and she'll obviously respect you more since you're a professional and she thinks I'm just some stupid bricklayer." In addition to not getting his concrete needs for information and validation met, he felt symbolically (and literally) castrated. With further discussion, Mike recognized that he was entitled to have his own views attended to, and that his job description had nothing to do with his inherent rights as a person or a patient. In a very concrete way, he was prepared to approach his psychiatrist again, tell her that this issue was very important to him, and ask for an immediate referral to the hospital urologist.

After this session, the therapist brought up this issue during the next treatment team meeting. She presented what Mike told her, and asked for clarification about "what really happened." Again, the therapist felt that she would have to proceed carefully in order to gather the appropriate information and to not ostracize the psychiatrist and promote even greater difficulties for her patient in the future. To the therapist's surprise, the psychiatrist responded unabashedly, "Oh, yes, I remember that ... he's the little guy with dark hair.... I don't see why he needs a referral now, anyway.... He's not married and he doesn't even have a serious girlfriend ... he doesn't need that problem treated right now; he's got more important things to work on." The occupational therapist on the team quipped, "So what if he doesn't have a serious girlfriend! It's his body and if he wants it to work right, why can't he get a referral?... Maybe he likes having one night stands or he likes to 'take care of things himself' but that's not any of our business to judge him."

To her credit, a lively discussion ensued in which the psychiatrist acknowledged that her cultural and religious views prevented her from seeing the importance of being able to achieve erection and climax, even without the promise of a steady partner. Mike's therapist also was able to articulate that his loss of potency resonated painfully with his overall feelings of passivity and hopelessness. The fact that his psychiatrist dismissed his concerns so easily also reinforced his feelings that he had no sense of agency or worth. The therapist then advised the psychiatrist to wait until Mike approached her to discuss the issue again (in order to provide him with positive reinforcement for a newly attempted, assertive behavior) before she made the appropriate referral. Working with the medical specialist, Mike and the psychiatrist then selected a different antidepressant medication that did not interfere with Mike's ability to have erections. Now that he was less preoccupied with his sexual functioning, Mike also was able to make more progress in therapy regarding his depression and more primitive defensive style.

Underlying Causes

Although it is vital for clinicians to address the psychological underpinnings of impotence, as a man ages it becomes more likely that the cause of his impotence is physiological (Galindo & Kaiser, 1995; Morley, Korenman, Mooradian, & Kaiser, 1987). Because the causes of impotence become multifactorial with age, educating and encouraging our patients to seek appropriate referrals becomes vital. Having a general knowledge base of specific illnesses known to lead to erectile difficulties can help to speed this process. The illnesses associated with impotence often include (e.g., Meston, 1997; Segraves & Segraves, 1995; Tsitouras & Alvarez, 1984):

- Diabetes mellitus. The vascular changes associated with diabetes, including a reduction in blood flow and circulation, can lead to difficulties in achieving erection. Neurological damage can also be associated with poor sexual function. Estimates suggest that up to 60% of male patients experience some form of sexual dysfunction within 5 years after the onset of type II diabetes (Schiavi & Rehman, 1995).
- Vascular disease including atherosclerosis, hypertension, sickle cell anemia, and Leriche syndrome. Plaque and occlusions in the blood vessels can extend from the coronary arteries to the penile arteries, making obtaining an erection difficult if not impossible. As noted in Chapter 5, other patients who have had heart attacks may fear the chest pain that often accompanies intercourse and limit their sexual activities.
- Endocrine and metabolic disorders such as hypothyroidism, hyperthyroidism, hypogonadism, hyperprolactinemia, Addison's disease, and Cushing's disease.

- Systemic disorders such as renal failure, myotonia dystrophia, and chronic obstructive pulmonary disease.
- Neurological disorders including multiple sclerosis, Parkinson's disease, temporal lobe epilepsy, Alzheimer's disease, stroke, pelvic nerve lesions, and spinal cord injuries.
- Substance abuse and dependence. Tobacco, alcohol, heroin, and cocaine have been shown to lead to difficulties in achieving erection and orgasm. Cirrhosis of the liver also has been associated with impotence.
- Pelvic surgeries that lead to damage of the neuromuscular bundle of the penis (the nerves and blood vessels that promote erections). Surgery to remove prostate gland tissue, colorectal surgery, and bladder surgery are typically responsible for such damage, even though procedures are being improved to avoid disrupting these nerves and vessels. Estimates suggest that removal of the prostate may cause impotence in up to 12% of all men who have this surgery (Schiavi & Rehman, 1995).
- Psychological disorders such as depression. Although it remains unclear to what extent impotence may be caused by psychological or physiological factors in this case, impotence and loss of libido are common symptoms of depression in older men.

Many older men and their partners feel relieved to learn that medical problems may be responsible for their impotence because most men attribute their inability to perform as a sign of personal failure or as a loss of their masculinity. Although many cases of impotence can be addressed primarily through medical means, many older men also display problems with sexual performance as a result of underlying psychological conflicts.

Widower's syndrome (e.g., Meston, 1997; Morley et al., 1987; Tsitouras & Alvarez, 1984) has been described as a commonly occurring phenomenon in which an older man finds himself unable to consummate a new marriage or relationship, even years after the death of his first wife. Unresolved issues of loss, grief, guilt about engaging in a new relationship, and fears of another painful personal loss are believed to manifest themselves psychosomatically and prevent the older widower from fully engaging in a new romantic relationship. For these widowers, individual psychotherapy and participation in support groups can provide an outlet for these feelings and thus unblock channels to future intimacy. As in younger men, general performance anxiety also can lead to sexual dysfunction. The use of sensate exercises, in which both partners have the freedom to explore sexual pleasure without the need to engage in actual intercourse, can alleviate such anxiety and reestablish psychological, as well as physiological, intimacy.

Side Effects of Medication

In addition to medical problems inducing sexual dysfunction, a number of prescription medications can induce impotence (e.g., Meston, 1997; Morley, 1996; Morley et al., 1987; Tsitouras & Alvarez, 1984). It is important to acknowledge that some physicians themselves are not aware of these side effects, nor do they assess the pros and cons of prescribing one medication versus another when the effects of impotence are particularly distressing for a male patient. Psychologists and other mental health care professionals can employ general knowledge of these medications to steer patients in the right direction for obtaining appropriate referrals and consults. See Table 10 for a listing of some of the more common medications that have been shown to produce impotence as a side effect.

Certain classes of medications, such as antihypertensives for high blood pressure, have been shown to produce some form of sexual dysfunction in

TABLE 10.  Prescription Medications
Known to Induce Impotence[a]

| Medication class | Drug | Generic or brand name |
| --- | --- | --- |
| Alpha blockers | Prazosin | Minipress |
| | Terazosin | Hytrin |
| Antianxiety | Benzodiazepines | Librium, Valium, Xanax |
| Antidepressants | Clomipramine | Anafranil |
| | Fluoxetine | Prozac |
| | Imipramine | Tofranil |
| | Paroxetine | Paxil |
| | Phenelzine | Nardil |
| | Sertraline | Zoloft |
| Antihypertensives | Clonidine | Catapres |
| | Chlorothiazide | Diuril |
| | Digoxin | Lanoxin |
| | Prazosin | Minipress |
| | Reserpine | Diupres |
| Antipsychotics | Chlorpromazine | Thorazine |
| | Clozapine | Clozaril |
| | Haloperidol | Haldol |
| | Mesoridazine | Serentil |
| | Thioridazine | Mellaril |
| | Trifluoperazine | Stelazine |
| Beta blockers | Propranolol | Inderal |
| Cardiovascular agents | Clofibrate | Atromid |
| | Digoxin | Lanoxin |
| | Disopyramide | Norpace |
| Chemotherapy agents | Various | |
| Diuretics | Chrlorothiazide | Diuril |
| | Chlorthalidone | Thalitone |
| | Spironolactone | |
| Hormones | Estrogen | Premarin |
| Mood stabilizers | Lithium | Lithonate, Eskalith |
| Parkinson's agents | Carbidopa/ levodopa | Sinemet |
| | Selegiline | Eldepryl |

[a]This listing is not comprehensive; a variety of other medications may cause similar effects.

almost all male patients (Morley et al., 1987). Up to 43% of male patients treated with hypertensive agents have complained of impotence (Bulpitt, Dollery, & Carne, 1974). Many medications that treat depression are implicated in the occurrence of impotence, although some antidepressants such as bupropion have been shown to produce less sexual dysfunction than others (Segraves & Segraves, 1995). Clinicians also should inquire about such sexual side effects; low rates of medication compliance have been attributed to the emergence of impotence as an unexpected side effect (Slag et al., 1983).

Ralph

Ralph was a 69-year-old man who was admitted to a psychiatric facility after being arrested for disorderly conduct. He had broken antennas off of parked cars after an alcohol-filled night out on the town. Ralph had been diagnosed with bipolar disorder and had apparently stopped taking his medication a month ago. He had become manic, unable to speak coherently because of pressured speech, and he manifested grandiose delusions and poor social judgment. Although he had a relatively high-paying job as a computer repairman, he spent most of his savings during the past few weeks on expensive clothing, dinners, and horse racing. His wife of 20 years threatened to leave him if he was not willing to stay in the hospital for extended treatment.

About 3 weeks after admission, Ralph had begun to make progress. He was prescribed lithium by the unit psychiatrist, and his mental status improved significantly. He still had some grandiose delusions, but his speech rate became normal and staff members could understand clearly what he was saying. Ralph was now able to plan for the future and recognize the consequences of his actions. He also had a healthy sense of humor and he used it to make friendly acquaintances with other patients. He participated actively in group and individual therapy, and the treatment team decided that he had made enough progress to have unrestricted visiting hours and run of the grounds during scheduled breaks.

The next week, however, a nursing assistant found Ralph sitting on a pool of blood on his bed around 4 a.m., clutching at his arm and hand. The window in his room had been broken, even though it was entwined with wire and sprayed with special coatings to make it impenetrable to all but the strongest blows. After receiving more than 35 stitches, Ralph was asked what had happened. Through pressured speech, he admitted that he had not taken all of his medication. When asked what had caused him to stop taking his pills as prescribed, Ralph stopped talking and stared straight ahead. He then lifted his arm above his head and screamed plaintively, "I can't masturbate anymore. I mean, I can't get off!... You can't take that away from me—even in this hell hole!"

Apparently, a side effect of the lithium prevented Ralph from experiencing orgasm; he described masturbating in his room "for hours" to no avail. "You have no idea how frustrating that is, you just don't know, especially for someone as important as me." What Ralph meant symbolically was that no one cared to recognize how important the functioning of his body was to him, particularly on a sexual level. Neither his psychiatrist nor psychologist had discussed impotence with him as a potential side effect of his medication, nor had they asked him directly about the presence of any such symptoms as he resumed taking his medication. Although Ralph's psychologist certainly was not responsible for his medication directly, the application of her knowledge in this area would have been quite relevant. If these professionals had intervened, or even made an appropriate inquiry, Ralph's serious injury could probably have been avoided.

## TREATMENTS FOR IMPOTENCE

A number of treatments are available for older men experiencing impotence. They generally fall into two categories: medical and psychological approaches. As noted, impotence among older men rarely has one underlying cause. Instead, the causes are typically multidimensional, and may include multiple medical problems or some combination of medical and psychological difficulties. Clinicians must be careful to avoid assuming that impotence is caused specifically by one problem or another. The current tendency appears to be the medicalization of impotence in which psychological factors tend to be downplayed or ignored (Rosen, 1996; Schiavi, 1996). This trend appears to be heightened further with recent advances in oral medications.

### Medical Approaches

Medical treatments for impotence can be grouped into three primary categories: vacuum devices, penile implants, and both injection and oral vasoactive drugs (Galindo & Kaiser, 1995). Each has its own degree of invasiveness, effectiveness, monetary cost, and observed rates of compliance.

Vacuum devices appear to be most effective in cases in which vascular problems underlie impotence (Galindo & Kaiser, 1995), and moderately effective for impotence related to diabetes and neurological disorders (Heller, Keren, Aloni, & Davidoff, 1992; Korenman & Viosca, 1992). A physician can prescribe the use of one of eight FDA approved vacuum devices (Gregoire, 1992) at a cost between $200 and $400 (Galindo & Kaiser, 1995). Essentially, a cylinder is placed over the penis and a vacuum draws blood into the organ to create an erection. A clamp or band is then placed at the base of the penis to maintain the engorgement of blood and its rigidity. Patient education appears critical; some side effects from the use of vacuum devices include bruising, numbness, and painful ejaculation. From a psychological perspective, many men are hesitant to use these pumps because they appear invasive and artificial (Meinhardt, Lycklama a Nijeholt, Kropman, & Zwartendijk, 1993), and because they are unable to hide its use from their partner.

In cases of spinal cord injury, severe vascular or neurological disease, or when all other approaches have failed (Galindo & Kaiser, 1995), penile implant surgery may be recommended. These procedures are costly, and range from $3000 to $5000. Silicone- or saline-filled rods are inserted in the penis; some require inflation for erection to take place. A number of problems have been reported following such procedures. These include complications from anesthesia, scarring, and problems in operating the device. If a device malfunctions and has to be removed, the odds of impotence occurring as a result also are relatively high (Galindo & Kaiser, 1995). Middle-aged men have reported greater satisfaction with this procedure than older men (Collins & Kinder, 1984), perhaps because older men are more likely to experience postoperative infection and because older men may have difficulties operating inflatable or hydraulic devices as a result of possible sensory deficits. Because this procedure is so invasive, urologists recommend that patients undergo psychological treatment both before and after the procedure (Schover, 1989).

A third approach to treatment of impotence is through the use of drugs. Self-injected vasoactive drugs such as papaverine HCl, phentolamine mesylate, alprostadil, and prostaglandin E can produce an erection in as little as 5 minutes that can last as long as 30 to 60 minutes. A major problem with this approach is that few of these drugs are approved for penile use by the FDA. Other problems include cost (up to $20 per injection), burning and pain at the site of injection, and, rarely, bruising, prolonged erection, and liver malfunction. Because both a high level of manual dexterity and visual acuity are required for proper administration of these drugs (Galindo & Kaiser, 1995; Rosen, 1996), older men with arthritis or visual impairments may be unable to use this treatment. Some older men prefer this method over both penile prosthetics and vacuum pumps because they do not have to involve their partners in the treatment; they can maintain some level of "privacy" if they choose not to disclose their problem to their partner. Of course, it remains quite questionable whether this willingness to hide their problem from their partner is a sign of psychological health.

## "Miracle" Pills

The most recent medical advances in the treatment of impotence involve oral, prescription medications. These drugs, including sildenafil citrate or Viagra, have been touted as miracle pills because an older man with impotence can take a pill, and within ½ to 4 hours before intercourse have an erection with purportedly few side effects. Viagra, specifically, prolongs smooth muscle relaxation through the mediating effects of nitric oxide. Because a simple pill is required, no cumbersome equipment, surgery, or needles are involved, and a higher degree of privacy or secrecy can be maintained if the man so desires. The cost of the medication is somewhat prohibitive, but under a variety of circumstances, Medicaid will pay for its disbursement. (In contrast, a number of private insurance companies are refusing to pay for this relatively expensive treatment, stating that sexual intercourse at a certain age "is not medically necessary").

Unlike other medical means of treating impotence, Viagra appears effective in treating sexual dysfunction caused by a variety of underlying problems including vascular disease, hypertension, diabetes mellitus, pelvic surgery (e.g., removal of a diseased prostate), spinal cord injury, and most notably a number of drugs including antihypertensives, diuretics, antidepressants, and antipsychotics. Clinical studies by its manufacturer, Pfizer, suggest that over a 1-year period, 88% of patients taking the drug showed a significant improvement in sexual functioning. Specifically, 69% of men taking Viagra were able to have erections suitable for intercourse, compared with only 22% of men in the placebo group. On average, men taking Viagra reported having intercourse 5.9 times per month compared with men on a placebo who reported having intercourse 1.5 times per month. All male subjects responded similarly well regardless of their baseline functioning.

This new medication is not a miracle pill per se, however. "Sexual stimulation" is required in order for a man to obtain an erection; it remains unclear whether this stimulation can take the form of visual stimulation or whether direct physical stimulation is required. An important contraindication of the use of Viagra is that of heart disease requiring organic nitrates for treatment. Men taking organic nitrate in any form should not take Viagra. Anecdotal evidence exists that a number of deaths (from cardiac arrest or stroke) have occurred in men who took Viagra without supervision from a physician, who lied about their current medical status in order to receive the medication, or who took Viagra in conjunction with recreational drugs such as amphetamines and cocaine. Common side effects of the medication include headache, flushing, and stomach upset. Only one dose of the medication can be taken safely per day. Among older men, healthy men over the age of 65 showed a 40% greater concentration of Viagra in their blood plasma after use. It remains unclear whether older men are more likely to experience side effects compared to their younger counterparts.

## Psychological Approaches

Regardless of the medical interventions used to treat impotence, clinicians must remember that *none* of these approaches provide protection against sexually transmitted diseases. It often becomes the purview of mental health practitioners to educate patients about the consequences of engaging in high-risk behaviors, or in assisting them in ceasing their participation in particular high-risk behaviors (e.g., having unprotected sex with intravenous drug users or prostitutes). With few exceptions, most medical treatments do not call for psychological intervention, nor do they necessarily involve partner participation.

The use of so-called miracle drugs also presents unique issues regarding psychological care. Anecdotal evidence, including various lawsuits, suggests that the use of Viagra or other "pop up pills" has led to the end of relationships and marriages. For couples who have either ignored the topic of impotence or who have settled into a sexual relationship that does not typically include intercourse, the sudden emergence of the male partner's interest in and pursuit of sex can be upsetting, unsettling, and sometimes frightening. Even though a male partner may "be ready" for sex within half an hour, older women, in particular, often require a longer period of foreplay and additional lubrication in order to enjoy sexual intercourse without pain or discomfort. Miscommunication between partners can lead to different levels of expectation for both frequency and quality of sexual relations. Some women have claimed that their partners sought out younger women who were more likely to satisfy their newly discovered "sexual needs." Again, communication between partners, often aided by a trained professional, becomes necessary for both parties to resume and enjoy sexual relations.

More general, psychological approaches for dealing with impotence include desensitization in the form of sensate focus exercises (Masters & Johnson, 1970), anxiety reduction techniques, and general psychoeducation about sexuality and sexual performance. In many cases, fear of impotence can become just as crippling as impotence itself. In sensate exercises and anxiety reduction techniques, couples are typically prohibited from engaging in genital stimulation and intercourse. Couples are given homework assignments in which they are to massage each other, take a lingering bath or shower, and explore each other's bodies without touching or stimulating their genitals. It is believed that by distracting the male from his internalized expectations about what is successful, he can become sexually aroused and paradoxically experience an erection (Cranston-Cuebas & Barlow, 1990). Such sensate focus therapies have been accepted and used widely as an effective means of reducing impotence (Rosen & Leiblum, 1993), although little empirical evidence has been gathered to bolster its use (Rosen, 1996).

Other psychological treatments for impotence that have garnered more empirical support, particularly among older adults, include cognitive therapies that incorporate basic sex education. Sometimes simply identifying unrealistic expectations (Everaerd & Dekker, 1985; Munjack et al., 1984), highlighting normal age-related changes to the sexual response cycle (Goldman & Carrol, 1990; Wiley & Bortz, 1996), or disavowing the central role of the penis in bringing pleasure (e.g., Zilbergeld, 1992) allows couples to engage in more fulfilling sexual relations.

Fred

Fred was a 67-year-old man who believed that he should be able to achieve an erection and have sex with his wife at least two times a week. Mary, his wife of 43 years, agreed to come to couples therapy at the insistence of her husband. She did not quite understand why he asked her to come to "his sessions," since she believed that he had been coming to the geropsychology outpatient clinic for treatment of mild depression. She described their relationship as comfortable and easy going, and said that from the time they met at age 16, they "were destined to be sweethearts for life." Both husband and wife were community living and relatively free from illness. Fred did have mild hypertension, and his medication may have contributed to his inability to have erections consistently.

In one therapy session, Fred announced, "Last time I asked [my wife] if she was ready for her 'semi-annual,' she replied, 'Oh, you mean our annual semi?'" He took his wife's comment as an insult to his masculinity and a jab at his inability to consistently achieve erection. Fred thus felt compelled to try to have sex with her even more often to demonstrate his "abilities as a man," which further added to his performance anxiety. On discussion, he was quite relieved to learn that she did not base the quality of their sex life on his ability to penetrate her vaginally; she was quite happy to engage in vaginal intercourse on a more sporadic basis while maintaining their participation in foreplay and other activities. Mary also recognized that although her comment was "funny," it masked some of her previously unexpressed, angry feelings toward Fred. She had begun to feel "put upon" because Fred kept trying to initiate sex when she wasn't always ready or "in the mood ... just petting and watching television together in bed would have been good enough for me that night."

In conjunction with a referral to a urologist, the couple decided that Fred would experiment with Viagra in order to alleviate some of his concerns regarding impotence. One important issue that the couple was able to agree on in therapy was that Fred and Mary were both to agree on the use of the medication *before* Fred took it, and that Fred would be primarily responsible for initiating these discussions. Mary maintained that she was happy with Fred "the way he was," but that she understood if he wanted to try out this "new fangled medication ... heck, I guess it can't all be bad ... a little more fun never hurt anybody." Both Fred and Mary reported that they were able to "talk about this kind of thing" like they never had before, even when they were much younger. They both noted independently that "coming to the doctor" had helped them significantly because this topic was certainly not a topic of conversation among their friends.

## PROSTATE CANCER

As any responsible discussion of female sexuality includes a review of breast and cervical cancer, any responsible discussion of male sexuality must include information about prostate enlargement and cancer. Only within the past decade has increased and appropriate clinical attention been paid to these disorders of endemic proportions. Enlargement of the prostate gland, or benign prostatic hyperplasia (BPH), has been described as a symptom of viropause or manopause. Prompted by changes in testosterone levels, the majority of men can expect to experience BPH at some point in their lifetime. Autopsy studies of men over the age of 80 suggest that nearly 90% of all men from this age group present with an enlarged prostate (Boyle, 1994). Nearly one-fifth of all men in the United States can be expected to develop prostate cancer as a result of BPH. To add insult to injury, most treatments for BPH and prostate cancer (i.e., chemotherapy or surgical removal of part or all of the prostate gland) induce significant side effects such as pain and swelling, a frequent need for urination, and, most notably, impotence (Wasson et al., 1995).

In large part because of the increased attention paid to this commonly occurring disorder among older men, a variety of new treatments have been developed to combat BPH. These include coagulation therapies, laser therapy, and supporting or stintlike devices (Moon, 1996). Additional, more controversial therapies touted by some medical authorities include just "waiting it out" because the presence of BPH does not guarantee the emergence of prostate cancer (Wasson et al., 1995). Other treatments for prostate enlargement include the somewhat controversial use of vitamin and mineral supplements including zinc (e.g., Evans, 1980; Horton, 1984) and the more widely accepted use of alpha-adrenergic antagonists (e.g., the prescription drugs terazosin, doxazosin, and finasteride).

One of the most insidious barriers to appropriate diagnosis and treatment is the hesitation of older men to seek treatment for symptoms. Many older men do appear to recognize the symptoms associated with BPH, including frequent urination (particularly at night), painful urination, difficulty in stopping urination, incontinence, intense urges to urinate, urinary retention, and difficulties in achieving an erection. However, many older men fail to seek medical attention until their sex lives are affected. One 70-year-old man cited, "I don't care if I have to get up at night five times to go to the john. I just don't want my 'other functions' to start going, if you know what I mean." Another 66-year-old rationalized, "I heard that you can live with this for a long time…. I heard that when they cut it out you lose it anyway [become impotent], so what's the point in knowing if I have it?" A common fallacy exists that all treatments for the disorder involve a surgical "treatment" that apparently is worse than the disease itself.

Reflecting the narcissistic injury inherent in the disorder, an 81-year-old man retorted, "Who gives a shit anyway; I know I'm old. So I probably have it…. I don't need to have my nose rubbed in it, too." Because the most effective test for assessment of BPH appears to be a rectal examination, as compared to an antigen blood test (Lee & Oesterling, 1995), some men decline to see their physicians based on anxiety about this examination alone. Thus, misinformation, fear, and denial play a significant role in poor compliance with diagnostic protocols. The assistance of a mental health practitioner may be the key factor in allowing older men to cope with the anxiety surrounding both the screening procedures and the potentially impending diagnosis of BPH. Clinicians can also can be invaluable in assisting older men and their partners in gathering accurate information and reviewing various options for treatment.

## SUMMARY

A critical element of male issues in elderly sexuality is for both patients and practitioners to recognize that male sexuality encompasses significantly more than the number of times per month one has intercourse or a man's ability to have an erection. At the same time, clinicians must be sure to recognize that, despite popular stereotypes, most elderly men place a significant emphasis on their ability to have vaginal intercourse, and that any erectile difficulties should be taken seriously. Impotence is one of the most common sexual problems that older men experience, and clinicians can play a vital role in providing patients with the ability to seek appropriate medical consultations, to allay anxiety about diagnostic procedures, to manage psychological problems related to sexual dysfunction, to involve their partners in assessment and treatment, and to resolve identity issues related to sexual identity and prowess. Despite the medicalization of elderly male sexuality, mental health practitioners continue to have a pivotal role in providing the appropriate care and relief for our patients.

# 9

# Elderly Sexuality in Traditional and Nontraditional Relationships

*Elderly adults may express their sexuality within a variety of interpersonal paradigms including long-term marriage, gay or lesbian relationships, bisexual relationships, second (or third or fourth) marriages, affairs outside of marriage, and various dating arrangements. Just as older adults themselves are not stereotypically traditional, neither are their intimate relationships.*

More clinicians are finding themselves working with older adults who are involved in both traditional and nontraditional romantic relationships. Even the use of the words *traditional* and *nontraditional* is suggestive of the negative biases traditionally aired toward gay, lesbian, and cohabiting relationships outside of the context of long-term marriage. Patients must cope with these societal biases and stereotypes, and most clinicians themselves have probably not received much graduate training or education regarding these relationships, particularly within the context of elderly sexuality. Controversy also persists among clinicians and researchers regarding various issues such as the adoption of gay or bisexual identities later in life, particularly among women, and the existence and the impact of outside affairs within the context of long-term marriage.

## A PAUCITY OF RESEARCH

The paucity of empirical research in these vitally important areas compounds the difficulties inherent in working with older adults in various intimate relationships. Although some excellent studies exist regarding older homosexuals (e.g., Dorfman et al., 1995; Slusher, Mayer, & Dunkle, 1996) and elderly adults who date or live together instead of becoming married (Bulcroft & Bulcroft, 1991; von Sydow, 1995), they are few in number and have significant methodological limitations. For example, most research regarding elderly gay men and women has been generated from financially secure, well educated,

159

urban populations. Although these studies' findings are legitimate and add a wealth of information to our knowledge base about gay elderly sexuality, the selective samples and small sample sizes employed make it more difficult to generalize from these findings to other samples of gay elders who may be from different ethnic groups, from a lower socioeconomic status, or from a rural background. One cannot fault the researchers for their skewed samples, however. Because of fears about disclosure and anonymity, recruiting participants for these studies can be both difficult and expensive. Urban areas are among some of the more accommodating places to recruit "nontraditional" participants because of their more liberal and accepting climate, and simply because greater numbers of people are available in one place at one time.

Just as it appears dangerous to generalize from empirical studies about elderly sexuality within the context of more nontraditional relationships, generalizing from clinical anecdotes may be just as potentially damaging to patients. When faced with a lack of concrete information or ambiguous information, it is easy to make assumptions that one clinical case or presentation will be similar to another. Such inclinations are natural, as clinicians (and patients) want to avoid ambiguity and feelings of inadequacy in response to incomplete information. A common defense against such feelings of loss of control is to rationalize and assume that one already has the knowledge needed to work with such patients. Another, equally damaging stance is to assume that if little knowledge is available about the topic, it must not be of much professional importance. Fortunately, such therapeutic work in these nontraditional areas of elderly sexuality can be among the most fulfilling and challenging, if clinicians can accept this lack of general empirical knowledge, and simply adopt the necessary focus on the patient's own, unique experience.

## OLDER GAYS AND LESBIANS

Despite the lack of multiple studies regarding older gay adults' experiences, general awareness of these elders' issues can be realized. Although they are one of the most neglected subgroups of elders, older gays and lesbians do comprise a significant proportion of the general aging population. In terms of demographics, estimates suggest that more than 3.5 million gay elders live in the United States (Gwenwald, 1984). Most researchers also are likely to warn that these numbers underestimate the actual numbers of homosexual elderly adults. Many gay adults, much less elderly gay adults, are reluctant to reveal their sexual identity to others for fear of derision, discrimination, or out of simple respect for their privacy (i.e., it is nobody's business whether I am gay or straight). For these reasons, among others, it remains virtually unknown what proportion of gay elders are among the institutionalized, oldest-old, or rural elderly.

The clinical issues among older and younger gay adults appear to have some similarities. Common themes have been described as: concerns about coming out to others; whether or not to affiliate with the gay community; the maintenance of meaningful, interpersonal relationships despite societal pressures to the contrary; familial conflicts including family secrets and parental guilt; difficulties with prohibitive religious beliefs; anxiety about HIV and AIDS, including fears of contraction and the loss of loved ones to the disease; fear of discrimination that may include fears of physical as well as emotional harm; concerns about available social supports such as informal friendship networks and formal organizations; and legal problems related to the exclusion of same sex marriage. Related legal issues recently have come to the fore in the gay community, particularly regarding a lack of shared insurance coverage, retirement benefits, and visitation rights.

Despite these similarities between the two age cohorts, important differences also appear to exist. Gerontologists suggest that, compared to their younger counterparts, gay elders:

- Are significantly less likely to receive vital information about HIV education, treatment, and prevention (see Chapter 6).
- Have fewer family members available to tend to arising instrumental needs, particularly regarding financial and health care support. Elderly gay adults do appear to gather significantly more social support from friendship networks than from family members, however (Dorfman et al., 1995).
- Are more likely to have children, grandchildren, spouses, and ex-spouses. Gay elders were raised in a generation in which one was supposed to ignore or put aside homosexual tendencies in order to ascribe to traditional family values and relationships. Thus, older gay adults are more likely to have married early in life or to have had children to "try to change" or to "do the right thing." The family dynamics involved have the potential to become challenging and, at worst, to become problematic.
- May have more difficulties forming informal social support groups or romantic relationships because they are less likely to easily identify one another out of concerns about revealing their homosexual identities to others. To compound this problem, few formal support groups or social organizations for gay elders are available outside of large urban areas (Slusher et al., 1996).
- May have been more likely to suffer greater persecution by the heterosexual community. In this elderly age cohort, gays who came out often suffered significant, negative consequences that included physical and emotional abuse at the hands of their predominantly prejudicial, heterosexual peers. The related clinical presentations of these unfortunate experiences in later adulthood could present themselves in later life as diffuse anxiety and somatic reactions to outright posttraumatic stress disorder.

Such issues can be expected to impact, both directly and indirectly, on a gay elder's sexuality. Clinicians must be aware that elderly gay and lesbian patients who present with concerns about sexual dysfunction in late life also are likely to be coping with more broadly based interpersonal and societal issues. Specifically, negative societal attitudes and pressures can be found, in some instances, to catalyze or even generate some of the problems associated with elderly sexuality. For example, one elderly gay man suddenly developed problems with impotence after his daughter (from a prior marriage in his early 20s) failed to ask both him and his partner of 18 years to an important family function. Recognizing that sexual dysfunction does not occur within a vacuum is essential in work with older gays and lesbians.

In working with gay elders, therapists must recognize that it is not appropriate to make any assumptions about their patients' attitudes, feelings, cognitions, family dynamics, or any aspect of their lifestyle (as in work with all of our patients). Issues certainly may arise regarding the therapist's knowledge or lack of knowledge about the gay culture his or her patient is from. Recognizing any such differences in knowledge often provides the first step in establishing trust and credibility between patient and therapist. Bridging the gap can be as simple as asking questions of a gay elder. Alternatively, therapists must be aware of their own countertransference and the role that it can play in such information gathering. Asking an elderly lesbian patient about her lifestyle, for example, should be accomplished with the conscious goal of increasing patient empathy and illuminating previously unresolved conflicts, but not with the conscious or unconscious goal of satisfying voyeuristic tendencies on the part of the therapist.

## Dispelling Myths Regarding Gay Elders

Historically, gay elders have been believed to be depressed, poor, and lonely (e.g., Dorfman et al., 1995; McDougall, 1993; Slusher et al., 1996). Logically, it follows that elderly adults in this condition would be either unable or unwilling to engage in meaningful or satisfying sexual relationships. In his classic article, Kelly (1977) outlined some of the specific stereotypes regarding gay elders, particularly elderly gay men. The myth of the older gay man is of a man who is obsessed with sex, particularly with younger men, but who is unable to develop an emotionally or physically satisfying long-term relationship with anyone. He purportedly rambles from gay bar to gay bar looking for one night stands while becoming increasingly depressed, unattractive, and fearful of being labeled as gay by other members of the community. The myth further states that the older gay male evolves into a paranoid, effeminate queen who seeks out friendships almost exclusively with heterosexuals.

The research findings regarding older gay men and women, however, dispel virtually all of these stereotypes and myths. In various samples, older gays have reported that while they may have some concerns about disclosure of their sexual orientation to others, particularly in occupational settings, the majority describe themselves as moderately involved in gay culture. The majority also report a moderate or high interest in sexual relations and a high level of satisfaction in current sexual relations, primarily with members of their own age group. There is no evidence to suggest that gay elders suddenly begin to seek out younger partners. Those elderly gay men and women who do not have sexual partners have cited the loss of a long-term partner, physical illness, or a conscious choice to avoid participation in a long-term relationship as the reason for their abstinence (e.g., Berger, 1980; Kelly, 1977; Raphael & Robinson, 1980). Other studies reveal that older gays and lesbians are not any more or less depressed (Dorfman, 1995), or more or less obsessed with their appearance than their heterosexual counterparts (Kelly, 1977).

Contrary to popular belief, some theorists suggest that the developmental and demographic changes associated with aging may actually work to the advantage of gay elders (e.g., McDougall, 1993). In our current society, it is much more acceptable for two older men or older women to live together as roommates or purchase a house than it is for a younger, same sex couple. It seems that society's recognition that people want and need companionship, coupled with its ageist assumptions that older adults do not engage in sex and that older gays and lesbians do not even exist as a group (because older single people must naturally be widowed or divorced), allows older same-sex couples to live together without causing any undue distress or homophobic anxiety among heterosexual members of the community. Because older adults in general are falsely assumed to be in poor health, heterosexual members of the community also do not appear to consider homosexuality as an issue when they see two older women or two older men walking arm in arm as they are ostensibly "just helping each other out."

Additionally, many segments of society assume that aging homosexual adults are physically disabled (i.e., harmless) and that they do not pose the same psychological threat as younger gay adults. This bias actually may benefit older gays in some respects. For example, one 68-year-old gay patient from a rural outpatient treatment program cited, "I love being old now! No one bothers me or my lover anymore, even if we sit close when we go out walking or out to eat at [the diner]. It's like they think we have run out of steam or something, and that no one will bother us because we certainly can't bother them.... I wish it was this simple when we were younger." Another elderly lesbian patient mused, "When [Lauren] and I bought our house together 20 years ago at 45 and 42, a few people in the neighborhood gave us a hard time. Nothing that bad, but no welcome wagon or cookies for us, either. But now that we're older, it's like the neighbors know that we are there for them if their grandchildren fall off their bikes and need someone to look after them. I think they like that we are good neighbors who don't throw wild parties and play loud music.... I wouldn't say we are everyone's favorite, but compared to some of the rough ones down the street, they could care less anymore if we are two older lesbians or not." Another elderly woman stated, "I guess I don't even look like a [stereotypical] lesbian anymore. No one looks at me twice with my short hair and lack of makeup. No one expects some old woman to dress to the nines anymore. So, I can really blend in if I want to."

Other theorists posit that because gay elders have had to overcome many obstacles in their younger days, compared to their heterosexual counterparts living in mainstream society, they already possess a variety of effective coping skills that allow them to adjust more easily to the challenges often associated with aging (Berger, 1982). Many heterosexuals cite discrimination as one of the most distressing aspects of aging, and because homosexual men and women faced such intense prejudice at an early age, they may be better equipped to adapt to the prejudice inflicted on them as they become older themselves. Thus, they may better avoid internalizing negative self-views or succumbing to negative, self-fulfilling prophesies. Consistent with this theory, a qualitative analysis of narrative interviews with more than 100 participants suggested that elderly gays and lesbians often possess the following intra- and interpersonal strengths: a strong sense of independence and self-sufficiency; the establishment of interests outside of one's family and career; the ability to foster and preserve both romantic and nonromantic relationships; an increased sense of personal autonomy and inherent worth; the capacity to adjust to living with a stigmatized identity (Wolf, 1982); and demonstrated successes in mediating potential crises, as in coming out at an earlier age (Kimmel, 1978). Because many gay elders have engaged in less gender role stereotyping in their own lives, the typical need to adapt more flexible sex roles with aging also may be fulfilled more easily (Friend, 1980).

## Support Systems

Social support is an important aspect of life that allows someone to adjust more easily to life changes and crises. This function is no different among gay elders, who have been found to have similar levels of social support when compared to their heterosexual counterparts (Dorfman, Walters, Burke, Hardin, Karanek, Raphael, & Silverstein, 1995). One interesting difference between the two groups, however, was that gay elders garnered more social support from friends than family members. This finding may, at first, appear to represent a problem in family dynamics because, traditionally, family members are expected to provide more instrumental services (e.g., money, long-term care) than friends. However, gay elders may have a history of developing meaningful, supportive friendship networks because their own families were initially resistant to their sexual orientation. In this way, they may be better equipped to gather different types of social support from more than one source, when compared to typical heterosexual, elderly adults.

As an additional boon to gay elders who establish peer-related, social support networks, theorists suggest that friends may be a better source of social support than family members. Compared to family members, friends are more likely to engage gay elders in important life review discussions including difficult or sensitive topics such as personal disappointments, fears of aging, and current and prior sexual relationships (Lewittes, 1988). Friends also are more likely to offer support and friendship because "they want to," whereas family members may offer assistance because they feel obligated or expected to. It often is easier to accept help from someone who gives it freely than from someone who extends help only because of perceptions that he or she has to.

In order to facilitate such friendly social supports among gay elders, various support groups and programs have been implemented successfully (Slusher et al., 1996). Some of these nationally known support groups include SAGE in New York City, GLOE in San Francisco, and GLOW in Ann Arbor, Michigan. Although the vast majority of these groups are located exclusively in large cities, some older gays and their therapists have formed support groups in suburban and rural areas through the use of local papers, local gay bars, and the Internet. Important suggestions for establishing and maintaining such a group include selecting a sexually neutral (i.e., not an exclusively "gay") locale, emphasizing social support as well as patient education, incorporating food and drink in the meeting to make it feel less "clinical," and providing sensitivity training for therapists and other staff members (Slusher et al., 1996).

## SEXUALITY AND LONG-TERM MARRIAGE

### Sexual Behavior, Intimacy, and Satisfaction

Another area that has received little attention from researchers and clinicians alike is that of intimacy and satisfaction in long-term marriage. Many studies have examined the predictors of divorce and discord in marriage, but few have investigated the predictors of marital satisfaction and fidelity in late life (Herman, 1994). A variety of factors have been associated with satisfaction in long-term marriage for both elderly men and women, including an internal locus of control (i.e., a sense of control and influence over one's marital relationship; Camp & Ganong, 1997), liking one's spouse as a person as well as a romantic partner, a long-term commitment to the marriage, agreement on common interests and goals, pride in one's partner and his or her achievements (Lauer, Lauer, & Kerr, 1990), and the ability to adopt more flexible roles as friend, nurturer, and caregiver (Siegel, 1982). This flexibility in social roles in later life is consistent with Gutmann's (1994) premise that older men and women have various opportunities to explore and adopt more androgynous sex roles. According to this belief, aging would elicit a more assertive sexual role among older wives, and a more nurturing role among older married husbands.

Although contrary to common myths and stereotypes, sexuality appears to be an additional predictor of marital satisfaction in later life. In a study of more than 100 elderly couples, over three-quarters of the respondents reported that they agreed on issues of sexual relations. Nearly 90% of the respondents reported that their sex lives "caused no problem or difference of opinion" in the last decade of their marriage, and that they at least kissed their spouse or shared some form of physical intimacy every day (Lauer et al., 1990). Other indicators suggest that although older married men and women engage in sexual intercourse less frequently than their younger counterparts, related primarily to the physical health of one or both partners, their level of satisfaction with their marriage remains similar (e.g., Herman, 1994). Thus, it becomes important to consider sexuality as a vital aspect of marital life, even in marriages that have lasted more than half a century.

Issues in Couples Therapy

Couples therapy for older adults essentially is similar between older and younger adults. Vital aspects for exploration often include how the couple relates as romantic partners and friends, how they divide responsibility for various chores and responsibilities at home, how they experience subjective feelings of love and emotional intimacy, how satisfied they are with sexual expression, to what degree they share activities and leisure time, and so on. However, because of differences in age cohorts, younger therapists may feel somewhat uncomfortable discussing issues related to sexual satisfaction and fidelity. Although the therapist's tendency may be to discuss those issues more gingerly, they comprise just as important a part of the couple's clinical assessment as in any work with younger couples. Even more importantly, this may be the first time the members of an elderly couple have been given the opportunity to openly discuss their sexual life, and their satisfaction and dissatisfaction with it.

The developmental challenges associated with aging also can pose some unique problems for older couples. These difficulties may be age or cohort related, and may include:

- Disagreements with adult children over money, wills, finances, or lifestyle choices
- Visitation rights with grandchildren, particularly if a divorce has introduced stepparents and step-grandparents
- The assumption of financial and emotional responsibility for grandchildren; anxiety about financial security, especially if on a fixed income
- A move to a new community or care facility
- Adjustment to a significant increase in leisure time or the loss of identity as a valued employee through retirement; the loss of friends and family members through illness or geographic relocation
- Adjustment to new roles as caregiver for a spouse who may be acutely or chronically ill

All of these changes and transitions can translate easily into sexual dysfunction or dissatisfaction.

Even though there is extensive pressure to medicalize elderly sexuality, clinicians cannot automatically assume that cessation of sexual activity is related to medical problems. Sometimes older adults internalize societal prohibitions against older people having sex or they may cease participation in sexual activity as a symptom of more serious problems in the marital relationship itself. In other words, although it is important to consider the origin of sexual dysfunction in older adult couples as a potential function of underlying medical problems and disability, clinicians must consider the impact of general societal pressures to avoid sexual contact in later life, and of deep-seated problems with intimacy in the marital relationship itself.

When conducting marital therapy with older adults, it also is vital to assume that an older couple's initial presentation may not be accurate. This is not meant to say that older adults are devious, mischievous, or lacking in insight; many older adults may present initially as a gentle, happy, loving couple because they were socialized to "be on their best behavior" when dealing with a professional. The notion of discussing family problems outside of the family unit appears foreign to many older adults, and may result in an initially positive, skewed presentation. In fact, many times couples do not initially seek out couples therapy. One member of the couple may present to a clinician with problems of depression, anxiety, or substance abuse, which leads to a trial of couples therapy. In addition, clinicians must not ascribe to stereotypes that older adults are "perfect or sweet" because they have stayed together for so long. Even though older couples do tend to remain married, compared to younger couples who are more likely to become divorced, older couples are just as likely to have serious problems in their relationships as many younger couples. For better or worse, older couples may be more likely to overlook (i.e., deny) or tolerate spousal substance abuse or infidelity in their relationship in order to remain married.

The Hortons

Don and Winny, 72 and 67 years old, respectively, arrived together at a treatment team meeting. Winny was excited that she was given permission to take her husband home from the Alzheimer's unit. Don had been misdiagnosed by a previous practitioner as having Alzheimer's disease, when in actuality he had a mild case of vascular dementia from sleep apnea. He could be maintained with an alarm monitor and oxygen supply at night, and his dementia was deemed mild enough for him to resume life with his wife at home. Winny beamed, "Oh, we love each other, and get along so well…. I can't wait to take my husband back home. Thank god!" The couple had been married for nearly 47 years and never reported any significant problems in their marriage.

Three weeks later, Winny suddenly came back to the hospital and wanted counseling because she "hates" her husband. She complained that Don was so upset that they had not had sex since he returned home, and she was furious about him "pawing all over me." When asked if anything else was bothering her, Winny exploded, "He drives me nuts! He wants me to do this, to do that. He tried to change the oil in the lawn tractor and dragged it all over the house and now I have to clean it up. And I have to make his favorite meals, and do the laundry. I am so sick of this!" With Winny's permission, the intake therapist consulted with members of Don's previous assessment team, and Don's original therapist was asked to engage the couple in marital therapy. The therapist's initial goal was to provide both Winny and Don with more education about Don's dementia and the changes that might follow in their relationship and household. Both parties also were educated about changes in sexual interest and response related to dementia.

During their second session, Don's sentiments mirrored those of Winny's:

"The woman makes me crazy. I try to do something, and I guess I don't do it quite right. She ends up screaming at me for something or other, no matter what I do. I can't take it anymore. I just want to be with her, you know. I'm her husband and I'm back home now." The therapist pursued the relationship between Don and Winny, and about the realistic and unrealistic expectations that each held regarding Don's cognitive abilities, and their mutual concerns about resuming sexual relations after his diagnosis. For some reason, the therapist felt that this discussion was falling on deaf ears, and neither party seemed open to discussing their feelings or fears about Don's mild dementia. The use of more concrete attempts to engage the couple in developing a homework assignment also appeared to fail.

Reasoning that Don and Winny's apparent lack of motivation masked some deeper problem, the therapist decided to take a different tact. In order to assess their prior conflicts and coping skills, the therapist asked, "What is the worst thing that has happened between the two of you—lately or in the life of your marriage?" Winny looked at the floor and began to tremble. Don said, "Well, I mean, I don't know.... I guess when I almost ran the mobile home off the road, right? I did have a few to drink, but ..." Winny interrupted, "Oh, yeah, you can't do shit right, can you Don? That's just it though, and you want me to just laugh and say, 'OK, that's all right,' isn't it?" Don's face contorted in anger and he leaned forward in his chair to invade her body space, "Yeah, just like you are always nagging, nagging, nagging! Goddamn woman. Don, do this. Don, do that. Don, don't touch me, blah, blah, blah, blah, blah."

The therapist turned to Winny, "What usually happens after Don talks to you like that?" Instead of Winny answering, Don blurted out, "Oh, I tell her, doc. I get right up in her face with my fist and tell her, 'I'm going to knock you a good one, woman, if you don't shut the hell up right now! I'm sick of your shit.' That usually shuts her up pretty good." Winny sunk in her chair, and Don started with a hmph and sat back confidently in his chair, staring at her. Immediately, the therapist established firm limits and boundaries, stating that violence, or even threats of physical violence, would never be tolerated and were completely unacceptable no matter what the time or circumstances. She informed Winny and Don that being upset and angry was a normal part of any couple's relationship, but that acting on those feelings with physical violence was completely unacceptable.

On further exploration, Winny indicated that Don rarely hit her, but that things "started getting worse" after his dementia was diagnosed and his impulse control had lessened. Dan hated feeling like Winny's "pathetic, can't do nothing right, child" instead of her husband, and his anger was expressed more and more often in inappropriate ways. It also appeared that Winny was accepting of Don's abuse over the years out of a sense of obligation and rationalization: "He never hit me in the face, and he always came home on time, didn't gamble, paid the bills, and never cheated on me ... and I do love him." The couples therapy took on a radically different direction when it was obvious that their lack of sexual satisfaction was related to more dire, underlying problems.

## COHABITATION AND SECOND MARRIAGES

Even though older adults are from an age cohort that espouses the virtues of marriage and committed relationships, older adults often elect to live together rather than legalize their relationship through marriage. Older couples may avoid marriage because of pressure from adult children who have concerns about loyalty to deceased parents or about potentially dwindling inheritances, out of respect for their first spouse who they promised, under god, to cherish forever, and out of practical concerns about income tax problems and estate planning. For those who do have second (or third or fourth) marriages, problems may arise regarding all of the above issues. In clinical work with both such married and cohabitating couples, it becomes vital to note the common intersection between the emotional and practical issues regarding their presenting problem.

### The Albertsons

Beverly Albertson, aged 67, was accompanied to the geriatric outpatient clinic by her husband, Dan, aged 71. Their marriage of 13 years was a second marriage (through divorce) for both of them. Beverly came to the clinic seeking therapy for major depression. She had lost interest in leisure activities, in seeing friends, in cooking, in eating, and in sex with her husband. Dan lamented that they once had been "very close," but that all of that activity had stopped over a year ago. Because Beverly and Dan did not appear to be well educated about depression, its origins, or treatment, couples therapy was proposed as an adjunct to Beverly's individual therapy.

During one couple's session, it became apparent that Beverly's depression emerged when she felt that things between them had so badly deteriorated that "it feels like there is no going back." When asked what she thought had happened, Beverly started to cry. Although Dan did not make any overt attempt to comfort her, he appeared anxious and distressed. Beverly continued, "I just don't feel special anymore.... He doesn't even touch me anymore. I don't even want him to touch me anymore. What for, anyway? I don't count. I don't matter to him, anyway. I'm just not worth anything to him anymore." When asked to illustrate a specific time in which she did not feel special, Beverly spent more than 15 minutes relating a story in which she and Dan went out to eat at a family-style pizza pub. Beverly would not even look at her husband when speaking.

BEVERLY: When he takes me out to eat there, we get the lunch buffet because it's cheaper. That's OK, and I can understand that, even though it's supposed to be like a date, or our special evening out. We don't have that much money between the two of us. But, he won't even let me order a soda. I can only get water unless I pay for the soda myself!

DAN: Beverly, we've been through this a hundred times! That's how they make all of their profit! They probably spend ten cents for that soda, and they get over a dollar from me! It's the principle of the thing. I want her to feel special, but it makes me sick to jack up their profit margin that much. I just can't do it. We can always get soda at home, so why do you have to have it when we go out?

BEVERLY:     But I want it. Why can't you just get it for me. It's one stupid soda!
DAN:     Well, it's one stupid dollar!
BEVERLY:     Well, maybe I'm worth one stupid dollar.
DAN:     Yes, but not when it goes in some scumbag, rich guy's pocket!

More of this continued and the situation escalated. The therapist allowed for the argument to continue because she wanted to observe their normal pattern of interaction during conflict. Beverly and Dan continued to bicker and yell. They turned physically away from each other, but crossed their arms on their chests in a similar way. Their therapist reasoned that despite their current dissatisfaction in the relationship, they still were connected, or at least unconsciously attuned, to one another.

BEVERLY:     Well, the last time [your daughter] came to visit, you sure as hell bought soda when we went out to eat!
DAN:     Well, she doesn't come to visit often from California, and I, I thought it was the right thing to do.
BEVERLY:     The right thing for WHO?

After both parties were instructed to calm down in order to process the interaction, Beverly was able to admit that she always felt as though she played second fiddle to Dan's daughter from his first marriage. She wanted to feel like she was his primary love, and that she did not have to compete to get his attention. More importantly, she was able to admit that she felt that Dan did not love her as much as his daughter. Her lips trembled when she said this, and on seeing her tears, Dan put his arm around his wife, reportedly for the first time in over three months. In a subsequent session, Dan also was able to admit that he felt like he was in constant competition with Beverly's first husband. He was a wealthy businessman who allowed Beverly to maintain a large investment account. He admitted that he felt upset because his retirement check could never compare with the kind of money Beverly had in her account. When asked why he called it "her account," Dan said that he felt slighted that she did not offer to have him as a cosigner in her financial dealings.

On the one hand, Dan said he felt he could understand Beverly's desire to maintain separate investment, savings, and checking accounts "for her children, for later, if something bad happened," but that he still felt disdained and overlooked. After all, Beverly did a lot of shopping and bought herself expensive clothes, and Dan lived off of his own, somewhat meager pension. Dan said, "I mean, one dollar is a lot for me, and it is nothing for her ... every time she asks me to spend that dollar, it's like ... it's like I'm just giving it back to her first husband or something."

In sum, physical intimacy for the Albertsons had become tied to one of the most troublesome aspects of marriage for couples of all ages—money. Specifically, the distribution of valued resources in the marriage appeared tied to perceived competition with spouses from previous marriages, actual responsibilities to children from prior marriages, and the absence of trust between partners. Only after concrete planning and decision making was made about the distribution of money in the marriage, including money that was shared and separate, were Beverly and Dan able to resolve issues of trust. Beverly was able to understand that Dan sometimes felt that because he rarely saw his daughter, buying her things was one of the ways he felt he could be connected to her.

Dan became able to understand that since Beverly's first husband had an affair prior to ending their relationship, she felt "safer" hoarding a sum of money in case her fears were realized and Dan decided he was going to leave her as well. Once Dan was able to set aside his competitive urges, to empathize with her fears, and to let her know that he *was* a *different* man than her first husband, Beverly was able to "share" more of her money in a joint account, and the couple began to feel secure enough in their relationship to engage in meaningful, satisfying sexual relations. (In a more symbolic display of their ability to trust and give pleasure to one another, they also began to order two sodas and pay for dinner out of their joint account on their excursions to the local pizza parlor.) More importantly, if the couple's therapist had pursued issues related only to their sexual dissatisfaction, the Albertsons' true, underlying problems related to their prior marriages would never have emerged.

## LIFESTYLE CHANGES ACROSS THE LIFE SPAN

### Demographic Changes

In the last few decades, a radical change has occurred in this country's demographics. Most pressing in the elderly population, the numbers of single older women vastly exceed the numbers of single older men. Specifically, single elderly women outnumber single elderly men at a ratio of nearly 2 to 1. A variety of reasons account for this large discrepancy in numbers. Women have a longer life span, and women from the current elderly cohort tended to marry men who were older than they were. Thus, women from the current elderly generation can expect to become widows at a relatively early age, and can expect to be widows for many years to come. As a result, the odds are stacked poorly against an older woman who wants to find an available single elderly male partner. On the contrary, opportunities for seeking available opposite-sex partners can be quite extensive for single elderly men.

### Adopting a Gay or Bisexual Orientation

A number of theorists have speculated that single heterosexual women may begin to adopt gay or bisexual orientations in late life in order to assuage their needs for an otherwise unavailable, male sexual partner. In terms of general economic principles of supply and demand, this adoption of a more flexible sexual orientation would appear to mediate the pervasive lack of available male heterosexual partners in later life (McDougall, 1993; von Sydow, 1995). Anecdotal stories of older women who develop such a homosexual or bisexual orientation in late life seem to abound, and often receive a great deal of attention in informal discussions of this topic. For example, one elderly woman remarked, "I really missed having a companion after my husband died. Judy and I do everything together now.... Sometimes we even sleep in the same bed and hold hands.... I really like having someone there." Unfortunately, empirical research regarding this phenomenon is practically nonexistent.

One pioneering survey of women between the ages of 50 and 91 years suggested that up to one third of their community-living sample "expressed interest" in women, but that only 4% actually engaged in recent homosexual activity. Further, the study found that those elderly women who did engage in a same-sex intimate relationship in later life had previous experience with homosexuality in adolescence or midlife. (It also is important to note that the majority of the elderly women who reported some lesbian activity throughout life reported having satisfying sexual relations with women.) In sum, these limited empirical indicators suggest that this notion of elderly heterosexual women blossoming into bisexuality in late life is not as common as perhaps believed. What is more likely is that younger lesbians who grew up in oppressive social conditions were unable to explore or express their orientation openly, and now have the proclivity or perceived freedom to do so in their advanced years. Ultimately, it appears vital that these theorists' hypotheses, although supported by general principles of "supply and demand" and some clinical anecdotes, may not represent the experience of the majority of older adult heterosexual women. Once again, it becomes essential to view each patient's case in the most unbiased and open-minded manner as possible.

Georgette

Georgette was an 87-year-old, twice-divorced woman who was seen in therapy for treatment of narcissistic personality disorder and major depression. She was a resident of a nursing home because arthritis now prevented her from tending to her activities of daily living, and because she had no immediate family members to tend to her daily care. Consistent with the external focus of someone suffering from narcissistic personality disorder, Georgette was obsessed with money, material possessions, and her appearance. Life review therapy allowed her therapist to initiate a trusting relationship with Georgette, and it assisted in important information gathering for an otherwise withholding reporter. More importantly, this work in therapy appeared to reduce Georgette's depression and anxiety.

In her course of life review, Georgette discussed at length her divorce from her second husband at 55. Although he was a wealthy businessman, Georgette managed to make him so angry that he refused to share his money with her (the court system at that time was not of much assistance). With what finances she did have, Georgette spent it on extravagant spa vacations and clothing instead of making any attempt to save for the future. At age 62, Georgette's best friend, Bette, took her in after she could hardly make the rent payments on her small garden apartment. Bette, a longtime friend from high school who lived in a nearby town, also liked to attend parties and other important social functions. In contrast to Georgette, Bette was a widow whose husband left her with a large estate and a massive inheritance. Georgette said that the two of them did everything together. "Bette was so terrific. She wanted me to have the best of everything, just like she had.... When we would go to the jewelry store, she always insisted on buying me something, too.... I wish I hadn't given that emerald necklace to my niece.... I always said 'no' to Bette about her buying me things like that, but she insisted that I have fun, too."

For more than 10 years Georgette and Bette lived in Bette's estate, each in separate rooms in her large residence. After a bout with heart disease, Bette passed away and left a sizable inheritance to her children and to Georgette. Although Georgette said that she was very sad and depressed when discussing her best friend's death in therapy, she did not shed any tears or appear overly distraught. On discussing the issue further, Georgette's therapist asked her if there was anything that she didn't like about Bette, noting that it was OK to have both good and bad feelings about the same person. Georgette became very quiet and said, "Well, there was that one day after the big party. I didn't like it.... I didn't like at all."

According to Georgette, one evening after a large social function, Bette had a few more cocktails than she had been accustomed. After all of the guests left, Bette followed Georgette into her bedroom and sat on the couch in the nearby sitting area. Georgette was sitting on the bed when Bette began to cry and talk about how much she missed having someone special in her life, and how much she liked having Georgette to talk to and to spend time with. Georgette said that she went over to sit next to Bette on the sofa and put Bette's head on her shoulder saying, "It's OK, friend. We have each other, right? Forget about those men!" A few seconds later, Georgette said that "Bette reached up—and grabbed my breast! I just stared at her and then I started screaming, 'What the hell are you doing? Get out of my room, right now! If you bring this up I'm leaving.' And, we never discussed it again." Georgette told her therapist that from that moment on "we just pretended that it never happened.... I decided it was still worth it for me to live there ... she was my best friend even if she was funny like that.... But it always did sort of bother me." Apparently, Bette felt trapped in a loveless marriage with her husband. She was a lesbian who had gotten married because it seemed to be her only option at the time.

Despite her narcissistic concerns and her obvious desire to remain in a situation in which her material needs were amply met, Georgette was able to process her confusion, fear, and anxiety about the entire incident in therapy. Her therapist worked carefully to assess whether Georgette had her own issues related to potential, latent homosexuality, and Georgette and her therapist felt that she did not have underlying homosexual tendencies. Through this discussion, Georgette also was able to move beyond her homophobic anxiety ("You mean it's OK to talk about all of this?") and recognize that Bette had faced significant adversity in her life; "It must have been awful to be married to someone, and have to sleep with them and do all of that, even if you didn't really want to…. It was bad enough for me when my husbands wanted to get in bed with me and I didn't want them to because I was mad at them or something." Georgette was able to acknowledge both her own discomfort at Bette's attempt to become intimate with her, and her own sorrow for Bette's unsuccessful search for romantic companionship. "That must have been lonely. I know I got lonely always trying to look for dates…. I guess it was a lot harder for her to look, too…. And then I never even wanted to talk about it."

Although Georgette never fully acknowledged her sometimes selfish reasons for living with Bette (she did admit that she might have wondered if Bette "liked her" when she bought her all of that expensive jewelry), she began to appreciate their friendship even more. She even recognized that, on some level, she was flattered by Bette's advance, but that out of unrealistic fears of becoming homosexual herself, she could hardly allow herself to consider it as a compliment at the time. Although Bette had passed away and could not benefit from Georgette's increased understanding and acceptance, Georgette's work in therapy allowed her to widen her acceptance of other people from various backgrounds who lived with her at the nursing home.

Dating among Heterosexuals

Recent trends suggest that older adults may be more likely to date versus marry and "settle down." This growth in numbers of older adults who are dating or living together is even recognized among savvy businesspeople as a burgeoning market, primarily because the dating behavior of older adults appears more varied than that of younger adults (Schewe & Balazs, 1992). Activities may range extensively from midnight walks, cooking, camping, and the opera to square dancing, art classes, movies, and exotic vacations. The pace at which older adults date and develop emotionally and sexually intimate relationships also appears faster than their younger counterparts. Although companionship appears to be the primary reason why older men and women seek romantic partners, studies suggest that up to 90% of the elderly people involved in dating report that love and sexuality play a significant role in their satisfaction in the relationship (Bulcroft & Bulcroft, 1991).

As noted, however, the virtual shortage of available elderly men has forced many elderly women to forgo dating, or to engage in a very competitive market. Those elderly women who do date often receive instant social prestige in their communities (McElhaney, 1992). Elderly women who date also tend to be healthier and more able to ambulate independently, whereas elderly men who date tend to be involved in social organizations and to own their own home. It remains unclear whether older adults who do date are more psychologically healthy than those who do not, or whether dating itself fosters the development of coping skills and life satisfaction (Bulcroft & Bulcroft, 1991).

Despite the apparent benefits of dating in later life, the virtual shortage of single elderly men has important interpersonal and instrumental implications.

One only has to visit a nursing home, retirement complex, or other older adult institution to begin to observe the underlying dynamics. One elderly man complained that his "dance card was always full," and that he never had a chance to relax with all "of those womenfolk around." Another elderly man's girlfriend laments, "Every time he goes out to walk the dog, the divorced woman in next unit asks if he would like to come over and have some coffee.... I can see that she's not wearing anything much under her housecoat, for goodness sake.... Sometimes it makes me feel very unsure about my relationship with [Raymond]. I mean, wherever we go, he's got women fawning all over him." Another single woman noted, "If I don't ask the men to go for coffee, I don't think they will be asking me. I might as well take a number before they get around to it."

For older women seeking male companionship, their socialization for dating included smiling innocently and perhaps flirting. Women from this generation were not supposed to ask a man to dinner or to their home; it was considered too forward. Many of these elderly single women must make tough choices about adopting different, more assertive roles and about engaging in more competitive relations with other women. For elderly women who may be living on a smaller, fixed income, having a male partner is seen as one of the primary means of establishing a more comfortable, financially secure lifestyle as well as a way of securing companionship and an outlet for sexual expression. One elderly patient proclaimed, "I need a man, or at least some kind of family. Who else is going to take care of me when I get older?"

### Justine

Dating can be difficult to accomplish, or even define, for some older adults. Justine was an 85-year-old, community-living widow of 8 years. She sought individual therapy for depression and for help in coping with problems related to her adult children. Her depression emerged soon after the death of husband, with whom she appeared to have a loving, caring relationship. Justine spoke candidly and warmly about their fun times in which they took warm baths together, walked in the rain (with umbrellas so they wouldn't catch colds), and dancing in the living room to their favorite old records. Justine and her husband also monopolized most of each other's time; they worked together in a family business and had few outside friends or interests. After 2 months into treatment, Justine had begun to mourn her husband's loss and to seek out other social contacts in her immediate neighborhood. For the first time, she began to get to know her neighbors. She also took a taxi to the local senior center twice a week and started to make some same-sex friends. Justine also admitted that although she had considered dating other men, her adult son seemed rather opposed to the idea: "You and dad were the perfect couple.... How could you ever top that?"

Approximately 1 month later, Justine's therapist began to worry about her patient's apparent change in mental status. Justine began to show significant signs of paranoia, and she described hiding things in her own apartment. She also talked about sneaking in and out of the apartment after "making sure that the coast was clear." Justine began to forget her appointments at the hairdresser, geriatrician, and ultimately with her therapist. Her therapist began to consider dementia or psychotic depression as possible rule outs for Justine, especially when she claimed that a man was following her to most of her appointments. Justine claimed that she did not forget about them; she just wanted to "go to them alone in peace!"

Because Justine either could not or would not describe anything about the man following her, it was assumed that her mental status was so impaired via dementia or delirium that she was recalling prior events improperly, or that she was so depressed that she began to create psychotic delusions in which she was the subject of romantic interest from another man. Her therapist scheduled a neuropsychology examination to rule out dementia and asked Justine's geriatrician to run additional tests to see if any underlying medical problems could account for her somewhat sudden change in mental status. The results of the neuropsychology testing were ambiguous. She was described as having only a mild memory impairment. Justine's geriatrician felt that she was quite healthy except for her arthritis, and that she was "just imagining things" to feel needed and important.

During her next appointment, Justine lamented that her mystery man had followed her to the hospital. Unwilling to ignore the possibility that Justine was relaying some aspect of truth in her convoluted stories, her therapist called security and asked Justine if she would go with her to the waiting room to see this man for herself. Justine hesitatingly complied, and when they turned the corner into the waiting area, an elderly man stood up with his cane and said buoyantly, "Justine, I thought you wouldn't be done yet! Can I walk you home?" After Justine's therapist was assured that her patient was in no immediate danger or physical threat from this man, they returned to discuss the issue in their session.

Justine admitted that she had been "keeping secrets ... that is my neighbor, Rob.... He can't get enough of me. He follows me everywhere.... Sometimes I like it and sometimes I don't.... It's nice because he helps me put my garbage out when it's heavy. He shovels my walk when it snows. He brings in my mail for me when it rains and helps me carry my groceries up the stairs. And, sometimes I just like having coffee and talking with him." Justine began to wring her hands and continued, "Of course, my son and ... his wife don't like it.... Rob's a married man. We, we haven't really DONE anything. Well, one time he tried to hold my hand and I pulled it away. But his wife sure is steamed. I'm afraid to come out of my house because one day she was waiting on her steps to yell at me and call me names.... I haven't really done anything, don't you think? I can't help it if he doesn't love her anymore, can I? He told me that she doesn't even bother to take a bath anymore or try to look nice. He gets tired of her nagging and moaning."

A number of sessions followed in which Justine was able to speak openly about her relationship with Rob, her fears about becoming emotionally involved with another man, her concerns about betraying her departed husband and son, and her feelings of ambiguity about getting involved with a married man. At one point, Justine considered a restraining order against Rob, but soon realized that she did enjoy his attention, even if it was a bit excessive. For the first time in 8 years, she felt "desirable and pretty ... like [she] was courting again." At the same time, she feared that her relationship with Rob would generate a storm of gossip in the neighborhood in which she "would never be able to make friends, with what all of the other women would think." Justine's therapist had to monitor her own countertransference carefully so that she did not interject her own beliefs about marriage and dating into the treatment dynamic.

Ultimately, Justine tried to speak to Rob and his wife about the nature of their relationship. She spelled out that she and Rob "were just friends because she didn't want to be responsible for breaking up anybody's marriage." Rob's wife remained angry about the relationship, and she forbade Rob to even speak to Justine. For whatever reasons, Rob's wife tolerated his lack of attention and did not appear to pursue a divorce, separation, or counseling. So, Justine continued their relationship under more clandestine circumstances. She felt that even though Rob had amorous intentions toward her, she did not act on them, making them "just friends, after all." Justine said she sometimes felt guilty about all of the time they spent together, but she rationalized it as "Rob's choice to make his wife angry; I didn't ask him to do any of this."

In the next few months of therapy, Justine also came to recognize that by being friends with Rob, she had selected a companion who could not, by definition, compete with her dearly beloved husband or upset her son because she "couldn't marry [him], anyway." Justine became better able to acknowledge her own needs for love and companionship, and she began to spend more afternoons at the local senior center in hopes of finding a single male companion. She appeared to recognize, on some level, that she wanted a relationship in which she took responsibility for her own actions and in which she did not have to hurt anybody else (i.e., Rob's wife). She also felt that she had been able to "say good-bye" to her husband, which allowed her to seek a genuine, romantic relationship, rather than a pseudofriendship. She also recognized that her son would have to come to accept her choice in companions; she was the one living alone without a spouse, not him. Like most of the elderly women in her situation, however, the only single men who went to the senior center already had a steady girlfriend.

## SUMMARY

Clinicians working with older adults can expect to encounter a wider variety of relationship issues than once thought. Older adults do date, have affairs, and have bisexual and homosexual relationships. Developmental issues associated with aging, including the influence of adult children, changes in lifestyle resulting from retirement or illness, and cohort differences (particularly regarding attitudes toward same-sex relationships, dating, and marriage), can be expected to influence an older adult's expression of sexuality. The virtual lack of single elderly men in recent demographic trends can be expected to play a significant role in relationship dynamics. Older adults also may be hesitant to announce their relationship problems early in therapy because of prohibitions about discussing family problems or secrets. Successful treatment begins with a trusting relationship and a willingness to overlook societal stereotypes on the part of both the patient and therapist. Looking for the larger issues often behind sexual dissatisfaction remains an essential part of treatment planning and assessment.

# 10

# Looking to the Future
# of Elderly Sexuality

*The field of elderly sexuality has already begun to establish its importance
as a clinical domain, but much room remains for progress, education, and
advocacy.*

## BABY BOOMERS APPROACH OLDER ADULTHOOD

When working with older patients, it becomes vital to consider that new cohorts, or age groups, of older adults are reaching their prime. These cohort
groups carry with them different social mores, expectations, and experiences
that can shape their clinical presentation. Because of exposure to different
historical events and general socioeconomic, political, and societal pressures,
for example, a woman born in 1900 would be expected to come from a very
different social culture, and may have very different attitudes toward sexuality
in late life than a woman born in 1940. In the next millennium, the cohort that
will become a major financial, political, and cultural presence is that of the
baby boomers. Understandably, their approach to and expectations for their own
elderly sexuality can be expected to be quite different from those of the cohorts
that came before them.

### Demographic Indicators

What defines a baby boomer? Demographers identify baby boomers as
people who were born between the years of 1946 and 1964, during the literal
baby boom produced when large numbers of American GIs returned home after
World War II. Many of these boomers grew up during good financial times, and
expected to live the proverbial American Dream. Although women often maintained traditional roles as young wives and mothers, as they approached midlife
they often attended college, entered the workplace, and established successful
careers outside of the home. Men in this cohort typically reaped great benefits

179

from secondary education and enjoyed job security for many years. The men and women from this cohort also experienced life-changing events such as the landing of men on the moon, an increase in expected life span through advances in medicine, the introduction of modern conveniences in the home such as television and the microwave, and the civil and women's rights movements. More relevant to clinicians, the numbers of baby boomers seen in therapists' offices can be expected to swell considerably. By the year 2000, nearly half of the baby boomers will turn 50. By the year 2011, the first baby boomers will reach age 65, or older adulthood. And, the overall increase in an individual's life span (e.g., an average of 73 years for men and 80 years for women; Ables et al., 1998) will continue to add a sizable number of older adults to our population.

In addition to this emergent increase in sheer numbers of older adults, baby boomers can be expected to have considerable impact on our country's financial and political makeup. Some lobbyist organizations such as AARP and certain political representatives have already begun to recognize the power of this large group of voters. Aging baby boomers have already expressed concerns about the viability of social security, Medicare's long-term care benefits, changes in health insurance policies, tax laws affecting retirement planning, and rules governing pension plans, as most can expect to live well into their late 70s or 80s. Businesspeople also are beginning to recognize the financial power of aging baby boomers as consumers. Contrary to popular myths, older adults, on the whole, are not poverty stricken, and baby boomers seem to dispel that myth even further. Older adults over the age of 50, who account for approximately 25% of the population, hold both the majority of this country's assets and its discretionary income (Bell, 1992).

A Media-Friendly Blitz

Within the next two decades, more changes in the general population and popular culture will begin to emerge in response to this growing cadre of baby boomers. More specifically, we can expect to encounter a media-friendly blitz toward older adults. Fortunately or unfortunately, this increase in positive media portrayals of older adults in the media will be motivated primarily by businesspeople who are interested in the baby boomers' enormous spending power (Bell, 1992). Compared to other, older cohorts who survived the Depression as youngsters and managed to carve out a living for a typically large family, many baby boomers benefitted from the country's economic boom when they were in their prime raising 2.5 children, while maintaining substantial savings and earning power late into life. In essence, baby boomers possess incredible amounts of disposable income relative to other age cohorts.

Advertisers know that the majority of baby boomers will be able to afford expensive drugs and health care services and products (e.g., Viagra, a rather costly drug treatment for impotence). Other businesspeople recognize that the aging baby boomers are a new consumer group who are willing to spend enormous amounts of money on products and services designed to prevent the signs of aging. Such markets include health clubs and personal trainers, vitamins and holistic medicines, low-fat foods, hair transplants, dietetic services, plastic surgeries, home exercise equipment, home security systems, and even girdles (aptly renamed "body shapers") and bras. Other emerging consumer markets for baby boomers include children's toys (i.e., gifts from doting grandparents), financial planners, second homes and retirement villas, and spa and vacation packages.

In order to entice baby boomers to buy their particular services and products, advertisers will begin to feature models and spokespersons who are elderly themselves. Older adults will be featured more frequently as models in print advertisements and television commercials, and as lead actors and actresses in television shows. According to basic principles of advertising, these older spokespeople will be selected primarily for their beauty and physical fitness. The older adults in these media portrayals also will be portrayed as intelligent, well spoken, popular, friendly, wealthy, and even sexy. Related to clinical concerns, these readily apparent changes in media presentations of older adults can expect to introduce some interesting changes in perceptions and expectations for older adults, and among older adults themselves.

## What Clinicians Can Expect

Although one might expect that all of these positive portrayals of older adults in these emerging media markets will lead to a decrease in negative stereotypes about older adults, the actual changes resulting from this media-friendly blitz may be less positive and even insidious. Because televised images are so quickly internalized as desirable prototypes in our culture, one might hope that younger generations develop more positive feelings about aging and older adults. However, additional, unrealistic expectations may be introduced because the positive portrays of older adults in the media are likely to be extreme and homogeneous. These biased images will show successful aging only as a function of "aging prevention," rather than an acceptance of aging and the successful integration of the changes that it can bring.

Among elderly adults themselves, these overly positive images may bolster already unrealistic expectations that they are to remain beautiful, youthful, and robust even if they encounter debilitating illness or experience a tragic personal or financial loss. Because older adults will not be represented in their full diversity in the media, elderly adults who are disabled, homebound, depressed, chronically physically ill, impoverished, or institutionalized will have no available role models, and may be more likely to look on their own personal situation with contempt and disgust. Thus, this use of vivacious, healthy, youthful elderly models and spokespeople may cause more problems for older adults than members of popular culture would like to admit. As clinicians, we can expect to see the impact of these and other societal and cohort changes in our offices.

When working with the new cohort of baby boomers regarding elderly sexuality, as compared to our current cohort of older adults, practitioners can expect to see some general differences in clinical problems and presentations.

Although the following certainly represent generalizations, a variety of cohort differences can be expected along these dimensions.

- Aging baby boomers will be more likely to seek out psychological treatment for sexual problems, as they grew up in a time when it was more acceptable to discuss sexuality among their peers. Compared to their older cohorts, baby boomers are more likely to have experienced and have begun to accept some aspects of a "therapy culture." They also are more likely to have taken psychology courses in college, to have read self-help books, and to expect sexual satisfaction as a part of life. This positivity, if realistic and accompanied by appropriate levels of patient motivation, can only be an asset in treatment. This interest in sexuality also will prompt more baby boomers to seek treatment for sexual dissatisfaction in midlife as well as in late life.
- Baby boomers will present more clinical issues related to underlying family dynamics. Compared to their older cohorts, baby boomers are more likely to cope with divorce proceedings, stepfamilies, second (or third and fourth) marriages, dating in later life, cohabitation, and poorly defined or overwhelming family caregiving responsibilities. This change in family structure, away from the core nuclear family, has the potential to introduce significant strain in intimate relationships. Sexual disturbances may emerge as an outward symptom of such underlying interpersonal problems.
- Higher rates of eating disorders and body image disturbances will be observed among both aging men and women in this cohort. One culprit for this expected increase in pathology is the internalization of artificially created media messages and images. The general directive in our current culture is to find the fountain of youth, "even if it kills you." Clinicians must be as willing to assess and diagnose the presence of an eating disorder or a problem in body image among their elderly, as well as their young adult, patients.
- Institutional elderly sexuality will become more prominent in clinical practice. Although the actual percentage of older adults who live full time in nursing homes or other institutions is small, as the sheer numbers of baby boomers increase as they age, the actual numbers of older adults in institutions will increase. Clinicians may find themselves serving as outside consultants or full-time staff members of such institutions.
- The medicalization of elderly sexuality can be expected to increase. Baby boomers grew up with a reliance on and respect for the medical profession. The baby boomers also had the benefit of "quick fixes" for many of life's problems through scientific and technological advancements. Thus, many members of this cohort will seek out seemingly quick and easy medical approaches for treatment of sexual dysfunction. Many may seek out a drug that may or may not be most effective in treating their sexual dysfunction. Clinicians also will need to learn to function effectively as interdisciplinary team members, and to emphasize education and appro-

priate communication with medical professionals between themselves and their patients.

- Aging baby boomers are more likely to show greater acceptance of alternative relationships in late life such as dating, cohabitation, interracial relationships, and both lifelong and emergent homosexual relationships. Although many members of this generation may continue to hold negativistic, stereotypical views toward such nontraditional relationships, clinicians are more likely to encounter patients dealing more openly with such issues in their own and in others' lives.
- The impact of less traditional gender roles on sexuality will become evident. For example, female baby boomers, compared to their own mothers, are more likely to have earned a college education and to have pursued a career outside of the home. These women may feel less obligated to fulfill a traditional wife's role, which includes directives to place her husband's sexual needs before her own. For aging male baby boomers, life after retirement often means having more flexibility to experiment with different sex roles. These men may assume more caregiving responsibilities (for either an ailing spouse or a young grandchild), seek greater variety in their leisure activities, and adopt more domestic chores about the home. Although such increases in role differentiation are seen as positive changes from a general psychological perspective, many older adults may not change as readily as their partner, or may feel threatened by their own changes in personal priorities and interests. These psychological pressures can certainly assert themselves within the context of elderly sexuality.
- More baby boomers will relate earlier experiences of sexual trauma in therapy, and will be more likely to recognize the possible connection between these earlier events and current sexual dysfunction or dissatisfaction. Members from this cohort are more likely to be willing to admit such sexual abuse, unlike prior generations who often felt that such atrocities were to be kept, for the sake of propriety, as a family secret. Clinicians will be able to benefit many older adults who will finally have an outlet to discuss such events and to process them accordingly. Clinicians also should be aware that older adults can experience rape or incest at *any* age and that in late life, older adults themselves may be victims *or* perpetrators.
- Computerized data bases will lead to greater access to information about elderly sexuality for aging baby boomers. This generation of baby boomers has become familiar with the computer, and older adults as a group spend as much or more time on the Internet than their younger counterparts. Clinicians also will be invaluable in helping aging baby boomers evaluate the accuracy of information they receive over these unregulated networks. The use of the Internet, via chat lines, also will allow many older adults to maintain personal connections if homebound, or to seek out others who experienced similar problems, resulting in a beneficial support network.

## THE NEED FOR INTERDISCIPLINARY PERSPECTIVES

The Medicalization of Elderly Sexuality

Another major change that can be expected in the future of elderly sexuality is the medicalization of elderly sexuality. In other words, the medical field may appear to take center stage in the assessment and treatment of elderly sexuality issues. In our current culture of fast food, fast transit, and fast forward on our VCRs, patients often want a "quick fix" in pill form. They may lean exclusively on medical treatments to remedy sexual dissatisfaction that really stems from underlying psychological problems such as marital discord, distortions in body image, or difficulties in adjusting to institutionalization or disability. Simultaneously, however, medical knowledge and expertise do play an essential role in helping older adults remedy many sexual problems; as mental health professionals we would be remiss to not educate our patients about their options. For example, all elderly male patients concerned about impotence should receive a medical consultation with a urologist or geriatrician in order to first rule out underlying medical problems. Thus, mental health practitioners will necessarily, if not preferably, find themselves enmeshed in this medical culture, and are likely to find themselves working extensively in interdisciplinary treatment teams.

Being informed from a variety of perspectives is the first step in functioning more effectively in such a requisite, interdisciplinary setting that is consistent with this model of medicalization. For example, knowing what a urologist can diagnose and prescribe, and what a therapist can accomplish in couples therapy can be used together to better aid an elderly couple coping with sexual dissatisfaction related to a husband's diabetes than can knowledge from either practitioner alone. This inclusion of medical treatment, or education of basic knowledge at a minimum, can allow patients to understand that some sexual problems are not "all in my head" or "all my fault." Clinicians also can aid their patients in developing more effective communication strategies when talking with their medical providers in order to get the best treatment and to ensure that their own interpersonal needs are met. This medicalization of elderly sexuality also has generated more research funding in both the private and public sectors for critical problems including impotence, breast cancer detection, and eating disorders among older adults.

Unfortunately, the medicalization of elderly sexuality also has a significant downside. Many patients and some medical professionals tend to take a unidimensional approach to elderly sexuality, in which psychological issues and treatments are devalued or dismissed entirely for the sake of a "quick fix" or pill. Physicians typically command higher patient fees than psychologists, and patients and physicians may see this monetary value as representative of the increased value of the medical treatment itself. Managed care companies, which tend to devalue psychological treatment, may be more likely to pay for a visit to a geriatrician or urologist than to a psychologist. Patients who rely on insurance plans also may be afraid to seek out treatment when they learn that their own insurance companies do not value elderly sexuality (e.g., certain managed care companies have said that they will not pay for Viagra drug treatments for impotence because "sex is not medically necessary" for older men).

As a mental health professional, the medicalization of elderly sexuality also is likely to evoke intensely negative countertransference. It can be very frustrating to value medical professionals' input, for the sake of best helping a patient, while those same medical professionals discard the effective treatments that you can offer in conjunction with, or in place of, theirs. As a result, many clinicians report feeling angry, isolated, inadequate, ambivalent, and demoralized. Other therapists fear that medical specialists will (sometimes quite literally) steal their patients after they make a requisite referral. In sum, the medicalization of elderly sexuality can represent a true narcissistic injury to even the well trained, established, and otherwise confident professional in the field. Interestingly, this phenomenon demonstrates in parallel process the experience of many of our own older adult patients as they are summarily and arbitrarily dismissed by other younger, privileged members of society. Fortunately, the incorporation of medical technology in the treatment of elderly sexuality also presents clinicians with opportunities for personal and professional growth, even if these opportunities are not immediately obvious.

## Working Effectively with Other Professionals

In an ideal scenario, clinicians will work within an interdisciplinary setting that incorporates professionals from a variety of disciplines including psychology, geriatric medicine, social work, psychiatry, nursing, and occupational and physical therapy. All of the professionals will work well together, with well-defined roles and proficiencies. No profession will be valued more than another, and team members will not feel territorial or defensive about consultations or treatment plans. Information about patients will be shared freely, and treatment team members will even arrive on time for scheduled meetings and consultations. Personality issues and conflicts will be kept outside of the treatment team dynamic. Sound too good to be true? Fortunately, clinicians are in a unique position to affect the makeup of a treatment team. Therapists are probably among the only team members who are trained in group dynamics, and able to recognize and analyze their own countertransference within such a group setting. Thus, a variety of problems are common when working within interdisciplinary teams, and therapists often have a unique opportunity, along with the often taxing responsibility, to address and attempt to rectify them.

One common problem experienced in group work is that the dynamics among team members may reflect the pathology of a particularly difficult patient. Similarly, the treatment team may act out its countertransference in response to a particularly difficult patient. This process may include the stereotyping of a group member or professional affiliation, or at worst, the denial of a patient's problems. Consider Irene, an 85-year-old patient who was acting out sexually in her nursing home. She repeatedly grabbed her crotch and exposed herself to other patients, staff members, and visitors. To make matters worse,

Irene had a severe personality disorder and would verbally abuse staff and treatment team members. During treatment team meetings, it always seemed that someone forgot to bring Irene's chart to the meeting. As a result, she tended to be the last patient to be discussed, with little time left for any meaningful discussion about her symptoms or treatment planning.

In such a situation, it can be helpful to ask treatment team members if they recognize a pattern in their response to a particular patient, and then to air their feelings about this patient. Many professionals from other disciplines may be pleasantly surprised to learn that having negative feelings about such a patient does not mean that they are insensitive, unprofessional, or unable to help that patient. Although excessive complaining and griping about a patient is not helpful (e.g., "nothing will ever help that old woman"), treatment team members can be encouraged to articulate and express their feelings appropriately, in a private group setting. After being validated by other professionals, some of the previously unexpressed anger and tension that stymied the group can be released, and more productive work can begin. This discussion of negative feelings about a patient also often allows the group members to move beyond their anger, and discuss underlying feelings of inadequacy and uncertainty about how to proceed.

A second common problem encountered is the dynamic in which one member of the treatment team becomes the group scapegoat or outcast. Motivated by frustration with patients' overwhelming problems, underlying anger at one person's limited professional skills, or jealousy over one member's apparent professional proficiency, team members may consciously or unconsciously select a scapegoat. Having one member of the group to project negative feelings onto allows other group members to satisfy desires for competition and aggression, and to enjoy enhanced feelings of proficiency and belonging. Unfortunately, this dynamic is not just distressing to the scapegoated member of the group. This dynamic operates to the detriment of open, egalitarian communication among team members that is necessary for effective treatment planning.

Sometimes simply highlighting the process or considering other reasons that the team members may be angry is enough to halt it. If reality testing shows that one team member truly is incompetent, this issue should be tackled directly but professionally for the sake of one's patients. To avoid future primal horde scenarios (e.g., Alford, 1995), leadership in the group can be rotated formally between meetings. All team members can be encouraged to comment on each patient's progress, and a devil's advocate can be assigned during each meeting to normalize the expression of opposing views.

A third problem experienced is that team members may become frustrated because their treatment plans are not followed, or because their treatment plans appear ineffective. In other words, the team may not be able to treat patients effectively because certain professionals or staff members are routinely excluded from the group. It is very common for nurses (in institutional settings, in particular) to be excluded from treatment team meetings or even from general communication with other professionals. It is not uncommon for nurses, who typically are overworked, underpaid, and underappreciated, to become angry and act out this anger toward other professionals who simply "give the orders" by not following the treatment plans that they "had nothing to do with."

In most cases, it becomes essential to include nurses, physical therapists, nutritionists, and even housekeepers, transportation workers, and cafeteria workers in treatment planning, or at least in patient information gathering. Making these professionals feel valued and appreciated goes a long way in ensuring that treatment plans are followed, and equally importantly, often provides an incredible amount of information that would be otherwise overlooked. Often spending even a few minutes to ask a nurse or orderly how a patient is doing lets her or him know that you value the patient and that you value her or his knowledge and expertise. At the very least, a degree of cohesion and teamwork can be established that leads to increased benefits for patients, as well as a more pleasant and familiar work environment.

A fourth, common problem in interdisciplinary settings is the establishment of a group pecking order and the establishment of professional leadership. Commonly, psychiatrists and other medical professionals are granted, or may simply take, a leadership role in the group. Other team members will have understandably different reactions to such an assumption of leadership. Some will prefer such a formalized structure, or may feel that because the psychiatrist is either paid the most, or has the most responsibility in terms of filing court papers, and the like, he or she is entitled to the leadership role. Other group members may resent the implication that leadership selection was made without input from members of the group, and that their professional expertise has been automatically devalued.

Sometimes such arbitrary leadership roles can be highlighted by problems on units themselves. For example, who has priority when appointments are to be scheduled? Can a physician interrupt a patient's therapy session without prior notice? Can a psychologist interrupt a nurse when he or she is busy readying a patient for bathing and breakfast? The delineation of professional roles and general respect for other professionals' tasks can help alleviate such problems. Sometimes simply apprising the leadership role, either through a majority vote, or at least through an open discussion of the institution's policy (e.g., physicians are automatically granted leadership) can minimize such inter-profession competition.

A fifth commonly experienced problem in group work involves generalized problems with limit setting. It can be very difficult to have effective treatment team meetings if half of the members saunter in 25 minutes late, if one team member asks the patient's family to arrive for a consult without alerting the other members, or if team members overstep their professional boundaries and begin to make recommendations outside of their area of expertise. Sometimes in outpatient treatment teams or consultation groups, one professional may submit insurance paperwork or diagnoses without discussing the possible outcomes (e.g., more or less visits approved, permanent diagnoses are placed in a patient's chart) with other treating professionals. These seemingly innocent or trivial mishaps can be among the most annoying to other group members, and lead to heightened levels of hostility.

As difficult as some of these boundary problems are to manage, they can only begin to be addressed by discussing the issues openly and with as little hostility as possible. Putting the offending party on the defensive, even though it may feel rather satisfying at the time, will only make matters worse. One approach is to state the problem, "I think it is very difficult to get through all of these patients within the hour when everyone arrives at different times. Does anyone else think so?... Maybe we can discuss another time that would be better for everyone, or suggest that those people who arrive late do more of the paperwork later?" Asking for input from other group members, avoiding the placement of blame on specific group members, and offering suggestions for ways to rectify the problem, as well as suggestions for providing consequences for negative outcomes can generate meaningful problem solving.

Positive Outcomes in Interdisciplinary Work

Although working in an interdisciplinary setting poses inherent problems, a host of positive outcomes can result for clinicians as well as their patients. One primary benefit of working as a member of a treatment team is the level of professional and personal support. Dealing with issues of elderly sexuality can be extremely taxing; there is relatively little empirical research to rely on, and the countertransference issues involved can occasionally be overwhelming. Working with patients on a daily basis also can be isolating, even in the presence of another human being. Having a colleague to share information with, to develop a multifaceted treatment team with, and to simply process a difficult day with, can be invaluable. Positive interactions with other professionals also can help prevent burnout, a common problem among clinicians. Sharing common concerns, excitements, and interests with another professional can be liberating and comforting.

In more concrete terms, the use of interdisciplinary teams also can lessen a clinician's liability risk. Just as having a psychiatric consultation for a suicidal patient can provide another viewpoint in a potentially critical situation, it also can provide some legal benefits. Sharing professional expertise in the realm of elderly sexuality, particularly regarding issues including anorexia and sexual victimization and abuse, can be just as valuable. Other reasons to seek out interdisciplinary relationships are that numbers of patient referrals can be increased among all professionals involved. Selecting colleagues for such a network must be done carefully to ensure that they have the same ethical standards and are willing to share in referrals and insurance paperwork responsibilities, but the professional and personal rewards can be well worth the effort.

## SUMMARY

Looking to the future of elderly sexuality presents clinicians with a variety of challenges and opportunities. Aging baby boomers, with their unique cohort experiences and resources, will pose somewhat different clinical issues than their older counterparts. The medicalization of elderly sexuality is likely to continue, and clinicians will probably find themselves working within interdisciplinary settings. Coping with treatment team dynamics also poses unique rewards and challenges in relation to elderly sexuality. Related to the increased emphasis on medicine in the treatment of elderly sexuality, private and managed care insurance plans may become interested in increased competence among professionals, including a possible certification in geropsychology. More research is likely to be funded and conducted in various areas including impotence, prostate cancer, breast cancer, the long-term effects of sexual trauma, eating disorders, and marital discord in late life. It is hoped that previously unexplored areas such as elderly sexuality among the oldest-old, minority group members, and gay and lesbian couples will gain increased clinical and research attention. Even though elderly sexuality is a relatively new field, its prominence and importance has emerged in time to assail many ageist, societal stereotypes and to properly assist a variety of patients. Clinicians are in a unique position to shape the future of elderly sexuality, and educating both our patients and ourselves represents the first step in this meaningful and distinguished process.

# References

Ables, N., Cooley, S., Deitch, I. M., Harper, M. S., Hinricksen, G., Lopez, M. A., & Molinari, V. A. (1998). What practitioners should know about working with older adults. *Professional Psychology: Research and Practice, 29*, 413–427.

Adams, M. A., Rojas-Comero, C., & Clayton, K. (1990). A small group education/intervention model for the well elderly: A challenge for educators. *Educational Gerontology, 16*, 601–608.

Albarran, J. W., & Bridger, S. (1997). Problems with providing education on resuming sexual activity after myocardial infarction: Developing written information for patients. *Intensive and Critical Care Nursing, 13*, 2–11.

Alford, C. F. (1995). The group as a whole or acting out as the missing leader? *International Journal of Group Psychotherapy, 45*, 125–142.

Allers, C. T. (1990). AIDS and the older adult. *The Gerontologist, 30*, 405–407.

American Academy of Neurology AIDS Task Force. (1991). Nomenclature and research case definitions for neurologic manifestations of human immunodeficiency virus-type 1 (HIV-1) infection. *Neurology, 41*, 778–785.

American Cancer Society. (1985). Survey of physicians' attitudes and practices in early cancer detection. *Cancer Journal for Clinicians, 35*, 197–213.

Apfel, R. J., Fox, M., Isberg, R. S., & Levine, A. R. (1984). Countertransference and transference in couple therapy: Treating sexual dysfunction in older couples. *Journal of Geriatric Psychiatry, 17*, 203–214.

Bachmann, G. A. (1988). Sexual dysfunction in postmenopausal women: The role of medical management. *Geriatrics, 43*, 79–83.

Bachmann, G. A. (1995). Influence of menopause on sexuality. *International Journal of Fertility, 40*, 16–22.

Badeau, D. (1995). Illness, disability, and sex in aging. *Sexuality and Disability, 13*, 219–237.

Bagley, C., Bolitho, F., & Bertrand, L. (1995). Mental health profiles, suicidal behavior, and community sexual assault in 2112 Canadian adolescents. *Crisis, 16*, 126–131.

Ballard, E. L. (1995). Attitudes, myths, and realities: Helping family and professional caregivers cope with sexuality in the Alzheimer's patient. *Sexuality and Disability, 13*, 255–270.

Barbach, L. (1996). Sexuality through menopause and beyond. *Menopause Management, 5*, 18–21.

Barile, L. A. (1997). Theories of menopause: Brief comparative synopsis. *Journal of Psychosocial Nursing, 35*, 36–39.

Barry, A., & Lippmann, S. B. (1990). Anorexia nervosa in males. *Postgraduate Medicine, 87*, 161–165.

Belchetz, P. E. (1994). Hormonal treatment of postmenopausal women. *New England Journal of Medicine, 330*, 1062–1071.

Bell, J. (1992). In search of a discourse on aging: The elderly on television. *The Gerontologist, 32*, 305–311.

Berger, R. M. (1980). Psychological adaptation of the older homosexual male. *Journal of Homosexuality, 5*, 161–175.

Berger, R. M. (1982). The unseen minority: Older gays and lesbians. *Social Work, 27*, 236–242.

Bernstein, N. R. (1990). Objective bodily damage: Disfigurement and dignity. In T. F. Cash & T.

Pruzinsky (Eds.), *Body images: Development, deviance, and change* (pp. 131–169). New York: Guilford Press.

Blum, H. P. (1973). The concept of erotized transference. *Journal of the American Psychoanalytic Association, 21*, 61–76.

Botwinick, J. (1984). *Aging and behavior* (3rd ed.). Berlin: Springer.

Bowman, E. S., & Markland, O. N. (1996). Psychodynamics and psychiatric diagnoses of pseudo-seizure subjects. *American Journal of Psychiatry, 153*, 57–63.

Boyle, P. (1994). New insights into the epidemiology and natural history of benign prostatic hyperplasia. *Progress in Clinical and Biological Research, 386*, 3–18.

Bradburn, N., & Sudman, S. (1979). *Improving interview method and questionnaire design*. San Francisco: Jossey-Bass.

Bretschneider, J. G., & McCoy, N. L. (1988). Sexual interest and behavior in healthy 80 to 102 year olds. *Archives of Sexual Behavior, 17*, 109–129.

Briggs, L. M. (1994). Sexual healing: Caring for patients recovering from myocardial infarction. *British Journal of Nursing, 3*, 837–842.

Brown, T. A., Cash, T. F., & Mikulka, P. J. (1990). Attitudinal body-image assessment: Factor analysis of the body-self relations questionnaire. *Journal of Personality Assessment, 55*, 134–144.

Buckingham, S. L., & Van Gorp, W. G. (1988). Essential knowledge about AIDS dementia. *Social Work, 33*, 112–115.

Bulcroft, R. A., & Bulcroft, K. A. (1991). The nature and functions of dating in later life. *Research on Aging, 13*, 244–260.

Bullough, V. (1976). *Sexual variance in society and history*. New York: Wiley.

Bulpitt, C. J., Dollery, C. T., & Carner, S. (1974). A symptom questionnaire for hypertensive patients. *Journal of Chronic Disability, 27*, 309–323.

Burgio, K. L., Locher, J. L., Goode, P. S., Hardin, J. M., McDowell, B. J., Dombrowski, M., & Candib, D. (1998). Behavioral vs drug treatment for urge urinary incontinence in older women. *Journal of the American Medical Association, 80*, 1994–2000.

Burrow, J. A. (1986). *The ages of man: A study in medieval writing and thought*. Oxford: Clarendon Press.

Butler, R. N. (1969). Age-ism: Another form of bigotry. *The Gerontologist, 9*, 243–246.

Butler, R. N., & Lewis, M. I. (1976). *Sex after sixty*. New York: Harper & Row.

Butler, R. N., Lewis, M. I., Hoffman, E., & Whitehead, E. D. (1994). Love and sex after 60: How physical changes affect intimate expression. *Geriatrics, 49*, 20–27.

Call, V., Sprecher, S., & Schwartz, P. (1995). The incidence and frequency of marital sex in a national sample. *Journal of Marriage and the Family, 57*, 639–653.

Camp, P. L., & Ganong, L. H. (1997). Locus of control and marital satisfaction in long term marriages. *Families in Society, 78*, 624–631.

Campbell, J. M., & Huff, M. S. (1995). Sexuality in the older woman. *Gerontology and Geriatrics Education, 16*, 71–81.

Carlson, H. E. (1980). Gynecomastia. *New England Journal of Medicine, 303*, 795-799.

Carolan, M. T. (1994). Beyond deficiency: Broadening the view of menopause. *The Journal of Applied Gerontology, 13*, 193–205.

Cash, T., Winstead, B., & Janda, L. (1986). The great American shape up. *Psychology Today, 20*, 30–37.

Catania, J. A., Gibson, D. R., Chitwood, D. D., & Coates, T. J. (1990). Methodological problems in AIDS behavioral research: Influences on measurement error and participation bias in studies of sexual behavior. *Psychological Bulletin, 108*, 339–362.

Catania, J. A., Turner, H., Kegeles, S. M., Stall, R.., Pollack, L., & Coates, T. J. (1989). Older Americans and AIDS: Transmission risks and primary prevention research needs. *The Gerontologist, 29*, 373–381.

Cawood, E. H., & Bancroft, J. (1996). Steroid hormones, the menopause, sexuality and well-being of women. *Psychological Medicine, 26*, 925–936.

Centers for Disease Control Update. (1995). Acquired immunodeficiency syndrome. *MMWR, 34*, 583–589.

Chrisler, J. C., & Ghiz, L. (1993). Body image issues of older women. *Women and Therapy, 14*, 67–75.

Cogen, R., & Steinman, W. (1990). Sexual function and practice in elderly men of lower socio-economic status. *The Journal of Family Practice, 31,* 162–166.

Collins, G. F., & Kinder, B. N. (1984). Adjustment following surgical implantation of a penile prosthesis: A critical overview. *Journal of Sex and Marital Therapy, 10,* 255–271.

Covey, H. C. (1989). Perceptions and attitudes toward sexuality of the elderly during the Middle Ages. *The Gerontologist, 29,* 93–100.

Cranston-Cuebas, M. A., & Barlow, D. H. (1990). Cognitive and affective contributions to sexual functioning. *Annual Review of Sex Research, 1,* 119–161.

Cummings, J. L. (1991). Behavioral complications of drug treatment of Parkinson's disease. *Journal of the American Geriatrics Society, 39,* 708–716.

Dail, P. W. (1988). Prime-time television portrayals of older adults in the context of family life. *The Gerontologist, 28,* 700–706.

Damrosch, S. P. (1984). Graduate nursing students' attitudes toward sexually active older persons. *The Gerontologist, 24,* 299–302.

Damrosch, S. P., & Fischman, S. H. (1985). Medical students' attitudes toward sexually active older persons. *Journal of the American Geriatrics Society, 33,* 852–855.

Davies, J. M., & Frawley, M. G. (1994). *Treating the adult survivor of childhood sexual abuse: A psychoanalytic perspective.* New York: Basic Books.

Deacon, S., Minichiello, V., & Plummer, D. (1995). Sexuality and older people: Revisiting the assumptions. *Educational Gerontology, 21,* 497–513.

Dietrich, A. J., O'Connor, G. T., Keller, A., Carney, P. A., Levy, D., & Whaley, F. S. (1992). Cancer: Improving early detection and prevention. A community practice randomized trial. *British Medical Journal, 304,* 687–691.

Diokno, A. C., Brock, B. M., Brown, M. B., & Herzog, A. R. (1986). Prevalence of urinary incontinence and other urologic symptoms in the non-institutionalized elderly. *Journal of Urology, 136,* 1022–1025.

Dorfman, R., Walters, K., Burke, P., Hardin, L., Karanek, R., Raphael, J., & Silverstein, E. (1995). Old, sad, and alone: The myth of the aging homosexual. *Journal of Gerontological Social Work, 24,* 29–44.

Dorgan, C. A. (Ed.). (1995). *Statistical record of health and medicine.* New York: Gage Research Inc.

Duffy, L. M. (1995). Sexual behavior and marital intimacy in Alzheimer's couples: A family theory perspective. *Sexuality and Disability, 13,* 239–254.

Eddy, D. M. (1989). Screening for breast cancer. *Annuals of Internal Medicine, 111,* 389–399.

Evans, G. W. (1980). Normal and abnormal zinc absorption in man and animals: The tryptophan connection. *Nutrition Reviews, 33,* 137–141.

Everaerd, W., & Dekker, J. (1985). Treatment of male sexual dysfunction: Sex therapy compared with systematic desensitization and rational emotive therapy. *Behavior Research and Therapy, 23,* 13–25.

Feil, N. (1995). When feelings become incontinent: Sexual behaviors in the resolution stage of life. *Sexuality and Disability, 13,* 271–282.

Fletcher, S. W., Morgan, T. M., O'Malley, M. S., Earp, J. L., & Degnan, D. (1989). Is breast self-examination predicted by knowledge, attitudes, beliefs, or sociodemographic characteristics? *American Journal of Preventive Medicine, 5,* 207–215.

Folstein, M., Folstein, S., & McHugh, P. (1975). Mini-Mental State: A practical method for grading the cognitive status of patients for the clinician. *Journal of Psychiatric Research, 12,* 189–198.

Fox, N. L. (1980). Sex in the nursing home? In H. Cox (Ed.), *Aging* (pp. 95–97). Guilford, CT: Dushkin.

Franzoi, S., & Shields, S. (1984). The body esteem scale: Multidimensional structure and sex differences in a college population. *Journal of Personality Assessment, 48,* 173–178.

Freedman, M. R., Rosenberg, S. J., & Schmaling, K. B. (1991). Childhood sexual abuse in patients with paradoxical vocal cord dysfunction. *The Journal of Nervous and Mental Disease, 179,* 295–298.

Freud, S. (1896). The aetiology of hysteria. In J. M. Masson, *The assault on truth: Freud's suppression of the seduction theory* (pp. 259–290). Middlesex, NJ: Penguin.

Freud, S. (1946). *Totem and taboo: Resemblances between the psychic lives of savages and neurotics* (A. A. Brill, Trans.). New York: Vintage. (Original work published 1913)

Friedrich, W. N., & Schafer, L. C. (1995). Somatic symptoms in sexually abused children. *Journal of Pediatric Psychology, 20,* 661–670.

Friend, R. A. (1980). GAYging: Adjustment and the older gay male. *Alternative Lifestyles, 3,* 231–248.

Fry, R. P., Beard, R. W., Crisp, A. H., & McGuigan, S. (1997). Sociopsychological factors in women with chronic pelvic pain with and without pelvic venous congestion. *Journal of Psychosomatic Research, 42,* 71–85.

Galindo, D., & Kaiser, F. E. (1995). Sexual health after 60. *Patient Care, 29,* 25–35.

Gardner, J., & Fonda, D. (1994). Urinary incontinence in the elderly. *Disability and Rehabilitation, 16,* 140–148.

George, L. K., & Weiler, S. J. (1981). Sexuality in middle and late life. *Archives of General Psychiatry, 38,* 919–923.

George, T. (1996). Women in a south Indian fishing village: Role identity, continuity, and the experience of menopause. *Health Care for Women International, 17,* 271–279.

Glass, J. C., Mustian, R. D., & Carter, L. R. (1986). Knowledge and attitudes of health care providers toward sexuality in the institutionalized elderly. *Educational Gerontology, 12,* 465–475.

Glass, J. C., & Webb, M. L. (1995). Health care educators' knowledge and attitudes regarding sexuality in the aged. *Educational Gerontology, 21,* 713–733.

Golan, O., & Chong, B. (1992). Sexuality and ageing: Some physical aspects. *Geriatrician, 11,* 10–11.

Goldman, A., & Carrol, J. L. (1990). Educational intervention as an adjunct to treatment of erectile dysfunction in older couples. *Journal of Sex and Marital Therapy, 16,* 127–141.

Greenwald, P., & Sondik, E. (1986). *Cancer control objectives for the nation: 1985–2000* (Monograph 2; Publication No. PHS 86-28880). Bethesda, MD: National Cancer Institute.

Gregoire, A. (1992). New treatments for erectile impotence. *British Journal of Psychiatry, 160,* 315–326.

Gupta, M. A., & Schork, N. J. (1993). Age-related concerns and body image: Possible future implications for eating disorders. *International Journal of Eating Disorders, 14,* 481–486.

Gutmann, D. (1994). *Reclaimed powers: Men and women in later life.* Evanston, IL:Northwestern University Press.

Gwenwald, M. (1984). The Sage model for serving older lesbians and gay men. *Journal of Social Work and Human Sexuality, 2,* 53–61.

Hebl, M. R., & Heatherton, T. F. (1998). The stigma of obesity in women: The difference is black and white. *Personality and Social Psychology Bulletin, 24,* 417–426.

Heller, L., Keren, O., Aloni, R., & Davidoff, G. (1992). An open trial of vacuum penile tumescence: Constriction therapy for neurological impotence. *Paraplegia, 30,* 550–553.

Hellerstein, H. K., & Friedman, E. H. (1970). Sexual activity and the post coronary patient. *Archives of Internal Medicine, 125,* 987–999.

Herman, S. M. (1994). Marital satisfaction in the elderly. *Gerontology and Geriatrics Education, 14,* 69–79.

Hillman, J. L. (1998). Health care providers knowledge about HIV induced dementia among older adults. *Sexuality and Disability, 16,* 181–192.

Hillman, J. L., & Stricker, G. (1994). A linkage of knowledge and attitudes toward elderly sexuality: Not necessarily a uniform relationship. *The Gerontologist, 34,* 256–260.

Hillman, J. L., & Stricker, G. (1996). College students' attitudes toward elderly sexuality: A two factor solution. *Canadian Journal on Aging, 15,* 543–558.

Hillman, J. L., & Stricker, G. (1998). Some issues in the assessment of HIV among older adults. *Psychotherapy, 35,* 483–489.

Hillman, J. L., Stricker, G., & Zweig, R. A. (1997). Clinical psychologists' judgments of older adult patients with character pathology: Implications for practice. *Professional Psychology: Research and Practice, 28,* 179–183.

HIV transmission in household settings—United States. (1994). *Morbidity and Mortality Weekly Report, 43*(19), 353–356.

Hobson, K. G. (1984). The effects of sexuality. *Health and Social Work, 9,* 25–35.

Hodson, D. S., & Skeen, P. (1994). Sexuality and aging: The hammerlock of myths. *The Journal of Applied Gerontology, 13,* 219–235.

Holmes, N. F., Fernandez, B., & Levy, J. K. (1989). Psychostimulant response in AIDS related complex patients. *Journal of Clinical Psychiatry, 56,* 5–8.

Horton, R. (1984). Benign prostatic hyperplasia: A disorder of androgen metabolism in the male. *Journal of the American Geriatric Society, 32,* 380–385.

Hsu, L. G., Crisp, A. H., & Harding, B. (1979). Outcome of anorexia nervosa? A prevalence study. *British Journal of Psychiatry, 128,* 549–554.

Hsu, L. G., & Zimmer, B. (1988). Eating disorders in old age. *International Journal of Eating Disorders, 7,* 133–138.

Hummert, M. L., Garstka, T. A., Shaner, J. L., & Strahm, S. (1995). Judgments about stereotypes of the elderly: Attitudes, age associations, and typicality ratings of young, middle-aged, and elderly adults. *Research on Aging, 17,* 168–189.

Ives, D. G., Lave, J. R., Traven, N. D., Schulz, R., & Kuller, L. H. (1996). Mammography and pap smear use by older rural women. *Public Health Reports, 111,* 244–250.

Jackson, H. O., & O'Neal, G. S. (1982). Dress and appearance responses to perceptions of aging. *Clothing and Textiles Research Journal, 12,* 8–15.

Janus, S. S., & Janus, C. L. (1993). *The Janus report on sexual behavior.* New York: Wiley.

Jonas, J. M., Pope, H. G., Hudson, J. I., & Satlin, A. (1984). Undiagnosed vomiting in an older women: Unsuspected bulimia. *American Journal of Psychiatry, 141,* 902–903.

Jones, J. (1994). Embodied meaning: Menopause and the change of life. *Social Work in Health Care, 19,* 43–65.

Kaas, M. J. (1981). Geriatric sexuality breakdown syndrome. *International Journal of Aging and Human Development, 13,* 71–77.

Kaiser, F. E. (1991). Sexuality and impotence in the aging man. *Clinical Geriatric Medicine, 7,* 63–72.

Kaiser, F. E. (1996). Sexuality in the elderly. *Geriatric Urology, 1,* 99–109.

Kaiser, F. E., & Morley, J. E. (1994). Gonadotropins, testosterone, and the aging male. *Neurobiology of Aging, 15,* 559–563.

Kaiser, F. E., Viosca, S. P., Morley, J. E., Mooradian, A. D., Davis, S. S., & Korenman, S. G. (1988). Impotence and aging: Clinical and hormonal factors. *Journal of the American Geriatrics Society, 36,* 511–519.

Kaiser, S. B., & Chandler, J. L. (1988). Audience responses to appearance codes: Old-age imagery in the media. *The Gerontologist, 28,* 692–699.

Kampen, D. L., & Sherwin, B. B. (1994). Estrogen use and verbal memory in healthy postmenopausal women. *Obstetrics and Gynecology, 83,* 979–983.

Kaye, R. A., & Markus, T. (1997). AIDS teaching should not be limited to the young. *USA Today Magazine, 126,* 50.

Kellett, J. (1991). Sexuality and the elderly. *Sexual and Marital Therapy, 6,* 147–155.

Kelly, J. (1977). The aging male homosexual: Myth and reality. *The Gerontologist, 17,* 328–332.

Kendig, N., & Adler, W. (1990). The implications of the acquired immunodeficiency syndrome for gerontology research and geriatric medicine. *Journal of Gerontology, 45,* M77–M81.

Kennedy, G. J., Hague, M., & Zarankin, B. (1997). Human sexuality in late life. *International Journal of Mental Health, 26,* 35–46.

Kernberg, O. F. (1991). Aggression and love in the relationship of the couple. In G. I. Fogel & W. A. Myers (Eds.), *Perversions and near-perversions in clinical practice: New psychoanalytic perspectives* (pp. 153–175). New Haven: Yale University Press.

Kimmel, D. C. (1978). Adult development and aging: A gay perspective. *Journal of Social Issues, 34,* 113–130.

Kinsey, A. C., Pomeroy, W. B., & Martin, C. E. (1948). *Sexual behavior in the human male.* Philadelphia: Saunders.

Kinsey, A. C., Pomeroy, W. B., Martin, C. E., & Gebhard, P. H. (1953). *Sexual behavior in the human female.* Philadelphia: Saunders.

Kinzl, J. F., Traweger, C., & Biebl, W. (1995). Family background and sexual abuse associated with somatization. *Psychotherapy and Psychosomatics, 64,* 82–87.

Knight, R. G., Godfrey, H. P., Shelton, E. J. (1988). The psychological deficits associated with Parkinson's disease. *Clinical Psychology Review, 8,* 391–410.

Korenman, S. G., & Viosca, S. P. (1992). Use of a vacuum tumescence device in the management of impotence in men with a history of penile implant or severe pelvic disease. *Journal of the American Geriatric Society, 40,* 61–64.

Kornhaber, B., & Malone, M. A. (1996). Creating a support group. In K. M. Nokes (Ed.), *HIV/AIDS and the older adult* (pp. 333–346). Washington, DC: Taylor & Francis.

Koster, A. (1991). Change-of-life anticipations, attitudes, and experiences among middle-aged Danish women. *Health Care for Women International, 12,* 1–113.

Kroll, J. (1993). *PTSD/borderlines in therapy: Finding the balance.* New York: Norton.

Kuypers, J. A., & Bengtson, V. L. (1973). Social breakdown and competence: A model of normal aging. *Human Development, 16,* 181–201.

Lauer, R. H., Lauer, J. C., & Kerr, S. T. (1990). The long term marriage: Perceptions of stability and satisfaction. *International Journal of Aging and Human Development, 31,* 189–195.

Lawton, M. P., & Brody, E. M. (1969). Assessment of older people: Self-maintaining and instrumental activities of daily living. *The Gerontologist, 9,* 179–186.

Lee, C. T., & Oesterling, J. E. (1995). Diagnostic markers of prostate cancer: Utility of prostate-specific antigen in diagnosis and staging. *Seminars in Surgical Oncology, 11,* 23–35.

Leiblum, S. R., & Rosen, R. C. (1989). *Principles and practice of sex therapy: Update for the 1990's.* New York: Guilford Press.

Lerner, A. J., Hedera, P., Koss, E., & Stuckey, J. (1997). Delirium in Alzheimer disease. *Alzheimer's Disease and Associated Disorders, 11,* 16–20.

Lester, E. P. (1985). The female analyst and the eroticized transference. *International Journal of Psycho-Analysis, 66,* 283–293.

Levine-Perkell, J. (1996). Caregiving issues. In K. M. Nokes (Ed.), *HIV/AIDS and the older adult* (pp. 333–346). Washington, DC: Taylor & Francis.

Lewittes, H. J. (1988). Just being friendly means a lot—Women, friendship, and aging. *Women and Health, 14,* 139–159.

Linsk, N. L. (1994). HIV and the elderly. *Families in Society, 75,* 362–372.

Lipton, S. A., Choi, Y. B., & Pan, Z. H. (1993). A redox-based mechanism for the neuroprotective and neurodestructive effects of nitric oxide and related nitrosocompounds. *Nature, 364,* 535–537.

Lipton, S. A., & Gendelman, H. E. (1995). Dementia associated with the acquired immunodeficiency syndrome. *New England Journal of Medicine, 332,* 934–940.

Love, R. R., Davis, J. E., Mundt, M., & Clark, C. (1997). Health promotion and screening services reported by older adult patients of urban primary care physicians. *The Journal of Family Practice, 45,* 142–150.

Ludeman, K. (1981). The sexuality of the older person: A review of the literature. *The Gerontologist, 21,* 203–205.

Makuc, D. M., Freid, V. M., & Kleinman, J. C. (1989). National trends in the use of preventive health care by women. *American Journal of Public Health, 79,* 21–26.

Malatesta, V., Chambless, D., Pollack, M., & Cantor, A. (1988). Widowhood, sexuality, and aging: A life span analysis. *Journal of Sex and Marital Therapy, 14,* 49–62.

Mapou, R. L., & Law, W. A. (1994). Neurobehavioral aspects of HIV disease and AIDS: An update. *Professional Psychology: Research and Practice, 25,* 132–141.

Marwill, S. L., Freund, K. M., & Barry, P. P. (1996). Patient factors associated with breast cancer screening among older women. *Journal of the American Geriatrics Society, 44,* 1210–1214.

Masters, W. H., & Johnson, V. E. (1966). *Human sexual response.* Boston: Little, Brown.

Masters, W. H., & Johnson, V. E. (1970). *Human sexual inadequacy.* Boston: Little, Brown.

Matthias, R. E., Lubben, J. E., Atchison, K. A., & Schweitzer, S. O. (1997). Sexual activity and satisfaction among very old adults: Results from a community-dwelling Medicare population survey. *The Gerontologist, 37,* 6–14.

Mattis, S. (1973). *Dementia Rating Scale.* Odessa, FL: Psychological Assessment Resources, Inc.

McCartney, J., Izeman, H., Rogers, D., & Cohen, N. (1987). Sexuality and the institutionalized elderly. *Journal of the American Geriatric Society, 35,* 331–333.

McCormack, K. A., Newman, D. K., Colling, J., & Pearson, B. D. (1992). A practice guideline for urinary incontinence: The challenge for nurses. *Urologic Nursing, 12,* 40–45.

McCormick, W. C., & Wood, R.W. (1992). Clinical decisions in the case of elderly persons with AIDS. *Journal of the American Geriatric Society, 40,* 917–921.

McDougall, G. J. (1993). Therapeutic issues with gay and lesbian elders. *Clinical Gerontologist, 14,* 45–57.

McElhaney, L. J. (1992). Dating and courtship in the later years. *Generations, 16,* 21–23.

McLean, A. H. (1994). What kind of love is this? *Sciences, 34,* 36–37.

Meinhardt, W., Lycklama a Nijeholt, A. A., Kropman, R. F., & Zwartendijk, J. (1993). The negative pressure device for erectile disorders: When does it fail? *Journal of Urology, 149,* 1285–1287.

Meston, C. M. (1997). Aging and sexuality in successful aging. *The Western Journal of Medicine, 167,* 285–290.

Meston, C. M., Trapnell, P. D., & Gorzalka, B. B. (1996). Ethnic and gender differences in sexuality: Variations in sexual behavior between Asian and non-Asian university students. *Archives of Sexual Behavior, 25,* 33–72.

Meyer, B. J., Russo, C., & Talbot, A. (1995). Discourse comprehension and problem solving: Decisions about the treatment of breast cancer by women across the life span. *Psychology and Aging, 10,* 84–103.

Monks, R. C. (1975). Sexuality and the elderly. *Canadian Welfare, 5,* 19–20.

Monteiro, W. O., Noshhirvani, H. F., Marks, I. M., & Lelliott, P. T. (1987). Anorgasmia from clomipramine in obsessive-compulsive disorder. *British Journal of Psychiatry, 151,* 107–112.

Moon, T. D. (1996). Management of benign prostatic hyperplasia. *Clinical Geriatrics, 4,* 23–46.

Morales, A. J., Nolan, J. J., Nelson, J. C., & Yen, S. S. (1994). Effects of replacement dose of dehydro-epiandrosterone in men and women of advancing aging. *Journal of Endocrinological Metabolism, 78,* 1360–1367.

Morisky, D. E., Fox, S. A., Murata, P. J., & Stein, J.A. (1989). The role of needs assessment in designing a community based mammography education program for urban women. *Health Education Research, 4,* 469–478.

Morley, J. E. (1996). Update on men's health: Progress in geriatrics. *Generations, 4,* 13–19.

Morley, J. E., Korenman, S. G., Mooradian, A. D., & Kaiser, F. E. (1987). UCLA geriatric grand rounds: Sexual dysfunction in the elderly male. *Journal of the American Geriatric Society, 35,* 1014–1022.

Mulligan, T., & Moss, C. R. (1991). Sexuality and aging in male veterans: A cross-sectional study of interest, ability, and activity. *Archives of Sexual Behavior, 20,* 17–25.

Munjack, D. J., Schlaks, A., Sanchez, V. C., Usigli, R., Zulueta, A., & Leonard, M. (1984). Rational-emotive therapy in the treatment of erectile failure: An initial study. *Journal of Sex and Marital Therapy, 10,* 170–175.

National Institutes of Health. (1993). NIH Consensus Development Panel on Impotence. *Journal of the American Medical Association, 270,* 83–90.

Nussbaum, J. F., & Robinson, J. D. (1984). Attitudes toward aging. *Communication Research Report, 1,* 21–27.

O'Brien, S. J., & Vertinsky, P. A. (1991). Unfit survivors: Exercise as a resource for aging women. *The Gerontologist, 31,* 347–357.

Paganini-Hill, A., & Henderson, V. W. (1994). Estrogen replacement and risk of Alzheimer's disease in women. *American Journal of Epidemiology, 140,* 256–261.

Palinkas, L. A., & Barrett-Connor, E. (1992). Estrogen use and depressive symptoms in post-menopausal women. *Obstetrics and Gynecology, 80,* 30–36.

Papadopoulos, C., Beaumont, C., Shelley, S., & Larrimore, P. (1983). Myocardial infarction and sexual activity of the female patient. *Archives of Internal Medicine, 143,* 1528–1530.

Pennix, B. W., van Tilburg, T., Kriegsman, D. M., Boeke, A. J., Deeg, D. J., & van Eijk, J. T. (1999). Social network, social support, and loneliness in older persons with different chronic diseases. *Journal of Aging and Health, 11,* 151–168.

Peterson, A. C., Levin, R., & Zweig, R. (1989). The erotized transference: An adaptive point of view. *Psychoanalysis and Psychotherapy, 7,* 129–141.

Petrovitch, H., Masaki, K., & Rodriguez, B. (1996). Update on women's health: Pros and cons of postmenopausal hormone replacement therapy. *Generations, 4,* 7–16.

Pfeiffer, E. (1977). Sexual behavior in old age. In E. W. Busse & E. Pfeiffer (Eds.), *Behavior and adaptation in later life*. Boston: Little, Brown, pp. 130–141.

Pfeiffer, E., & Davis, G. C. (1972). Determinants of sexual behavior in middle and old age. *Journal of the American Geriatric Society, 33*, 635–643.

Pizzi, E. R., & Wolf, Z. R. (1998). Health risks and health promotion for older women: Utility of a health promotion diary. *Holistic Nursing Practice, 2*, 62–68.

Pliner, P., Chaiken, S., & Flett, G. L. (1990). Gender differences in concern with body weight and physical appearance over the life span. *Personality and Social Psychology Bulletin, 16*, 263–273.

Plutchik, R., Conte, H., & Weiner, M. (1973). Studies of body image II: Dollar values of body parts. *Journal of Gerontology, 28*, 89–91.

Plutchik, R., Weiner, M., & Conte, H. (1971). Studies of body image I: Body worries and body discomforts. *Journal of Gerontology, 26*, 344–350.

Poggi, R. G., & Berland, D. I. (1985). The therapists' reactions to the elderly. *The Gerontologist, 25*, 508–513.

Porcino, J. (1985). Psychological aspects of aging in women. *Women and Health, 10*, 115–122.

Price, W. A., Gianni, A. J., & Colella, J. (1985). Anorexia nervosa in the elderly. *Journal of the American Geriatric Society, 33*, 213–215.

Rackley, J. V., Warren, S. A., & Bird, G. W. (1988). Determinants of body image in women at midlife. *Psychological Reports, 62*, 9–10.

Raphael, S., & Robinson, M. (1980). The older lesbian: Love relationships and friendship patterns. *Alternative Lifestyles, 3*, 207–229.

Rappaport, E. A. (1956). The management of an eroticized transference. *Psychoanalytic Quarterly, 25*, 515–529.

Rimer, B. K., Ross, E., Cristinzio, S., & King, E. (1992). Older women's participation in breast screening. *The Journal of Gerontology, 47*, 85–91.

Robinson, B. E., & Balducci, L. (1995). Breast lump in an 85 year old woman with dementia: A decision analysis. *Journal of the American Geriatric Society, 43*, 282–285.

Robinson, G. (1996). Cross-cultural perspectives on menopause. *The Journal of Nervous and Mental Disease, 184*, 453–458.

Rodin, J., Silberstein, L., & Streigel-Moore, R. (1984). Women and weight: A normative discontent. In *Nebraska Symposium on Motivation 1984* (pp. 267–304). Lincoln: University of Nebraska Press.

Ronch, J. L. (1985). Suspected anorexia nervosa in a 75 year old institutionalized male: Issues in diagnosis and intervention. *Clinical Gerontologist, 4*, 31–38.

Rosen, R. C. (1996). Erectile dysfunction: The medicalization of male sexuality. *Clinical Psychology Review, 16*, 497–519.

Rosen, R. C., & Leiblum, S. R. (1993). Treatment of male erectile disorders: Current options and dilemmas. *Journal of Sexual and Marital Therapy, 8*, 5–9.

Rosenzweig, R., & Fillit, H. (1992). Probable heterosexual transmission of AIDS in an aged woman. *Journal of the American Geriatric Society, 40*, 1261–1264.

Roughan, P. A., Kaiser, F. E., & Morley, J. E. (1993). Sexuality and the older woman. *Care of the Older Woman, 1*, 87–106.

Sbrocco, T., Weisberg, R. B., & Barlow, D. H. (1995). Sexual dysfunction in the older adult: Assessment of psychosocial factors. *Sexuality and Disability, 13*, 201–217.

Schewe, C. D., & Balazs, A. L. (1992). Role transitions in older adults: A marketing opportunity. *Psychology and Marketing, 9*, 85–99.

Schiavi, R. C. (1996). Sexuality and male aging: From performance to satisfaction. *Journal of Sex and Marital Therapy, 11*, 9–13.

Schiavi, R. C., & Rehman, J. (1995). Sexuality and aging. *Urologic Clinics of North America, 22*, 711–726.

Schiavi, R. C., Schreiner-Engel, P., White, D., & Mandeli, J. (1991). The relationship between pituitary–gonadal function and sexual behavior in healthy aging men. *Journal of Psychosomatic Medicine, 53*, 363–374.

Schiavi, R. C., & Segraves, R. T. (1995). The biology of sexual function. *Psychiatric Clinics of North America, 18*, 7–23.

Schover, L. R. (1989). Sex therapy for the penile prosthesis recipient. *Urologic Clinics of North America, 16*, 91–98.

Schulz, R., Williamson, G. M., & Bridges, M. (1991). *Limb amputation among the elderly: Psychosocial factors influencing treatment.* Washington, DC: AARP Andrus Foundation.

Scogin, F., & McElreath, L. (1994). Efficacy of psychosocial treatments for geriatric depression: A quantitative review. *Journal of Consulting and Clinical Psychology, 62*, 69–73.

Segraves, R. T., & Segraves, K. B. (1995). Human sexuality and aging. *Journal of Sex Education and Therapy, 21*, 88–102.

Seidl, A., Bullough, B., Haughey, B., Scherer, Y., Rhodes, M., & Brown, G. (1991). Understanding the effects of a myocardial infarction on sexual functioning: A basis for sexual counseling. *Rehabilitation Nursing, 16*, 255–265.

Siegel, R. J. (1982). The long term marriage: Implications for therapy. *Women and Therapy, 1*, 3–11.

Slag, M. F., Morley, J. E., Elson, M. K., Trence, D. L., Nelson, C. J., Nelson, A. E., Kinlaw, W. B., Beyer, H. S., Nuttall, F. Q., & Shafer, R. B. (1983). Impotence in medical clinic outpatients. *Journal of the American Medical Association, 249*, 1736–1740.

Slimmer, L. W. (1987). Perceptions of learned helplessness. *Journal of Gerontological Nursing, 13*, 33–37.

Slusher, M. P., Mayer, C. J., & Dunkle, R. E. (1996). Gays and lesbians older and wiser (GLOW): A support group for older gay people. *The Gerontologist, 36*, 118–123.

Smith, M. M., & Schmall, V. L. (1983). Knowledge and attitudes toward sexuality and sex education of a select group of older people. *Gerontology and Geriatrics Education, 3/4*, 259–269.

Solomon, K. (1996). Psychosocial issues. In K. M. Nokes (Ed.), *HIV/AIDS and the older adult* (pp. 333–346). Washington, DC: Taylor & Francis.

Starr, B. D., & Weiner, M. B. (1981). *The Starr–Weiner report on sex and sexuality in the mature years.* Briarcliff Manor, NY: Stein & Day.

Stone, L. (1977). *The family, sex, and marriage in England, 1500–1800.* New York: Harper & Row.

Szasz, G. (1983). Sexual incidents in an extended care unit for aged men. *Journal of the American Geriatric Society, 31*, 407–411.

Taylor, D. H., McPherson, K., Parbhoo, S., & Perry, N. (1996). Response of women aged 65–74 to invitation for screening for breast cancer by mammography: A pilot study in London, UK. *Journal of Epidemiology and Community Health, 50*, 77–80.

Theander, S. (1985). Outcome and prognosis in anorexia nervosa and bulimia: Some results of previous investigations, compared with those of a Swedish long-term study. *Journal of Psychiatric Research, 19*, 493–508.

Thirlaway, K., Fallowfield, L., & Cuzick, J. (1996). The sexual activity questionnaire: A measure of women's sexual functioning. *Quality of Life Research, 5*, 81–90.

Thompson, D. (1990). Intercourse after myocardial infarction. *Nursing Standard, 4*, 32–33.

Tsitouras, P. D., & Alvarez, R. R. (1984). Etiology and management of sexual dysfunction in elderly men. *Psychiatric Medicine, 2*, 43–55.

Unger, A. K. (1985). Movement therapy for the geriatric population. *Clinical Gerontologist, 3*, 46–47.

U.S. Bureau of the Census (1993). *We the American elderly* (93-0626-P WE-9). Washington, DC: U.S. Government Printing Office.

U.S. Bureau of the Census. (1996). *65+ in the United States* (Current Population Reports, Special Studies, P23-190). Washington, DC: U.S. Government Printing Office.

Van Deusen, J. (1997). Body image of non-clinical and clinical populations of men: A literature review. *Occupational Therapy in Mental Health, 13*, 37–57.

Voda, A. M., Christy, N. S., & Morgan, J. M. (1991). Body composition changes in menopausal women. *Women and Therapy, 11*, 71–96.

von Sydow, K. (1995). Unconventional sexual relationships: Data about German women ages 50 to 91 years. *Archives of Sexual Behavior, 24*, 271–283.

Wade, D. T., & Hewer, R. L. (1985). Outlook after an acute stroke: Urinary incontinence and loss of consciousness in 532 patients. *Quarterly Journal of Medicine, 56*, 601–608.

Walker, B. L., Osgood, N. J., Richardson, J. P., & Ephross, P. H. (1998). Staff and elderly knowledge and attitudes toward elderly sexuality. *Educational Gerontology, 24*, 471–489.

Walker, P. W., Cole, J. O., Gardner, E. A., Hughes, A. R., Johnston, J. A., Batey, S. R., & Lineberry, C. G.

(1993). Improvement in fluoxetine-associated sexual dysfunction in patients switched to bupropion. *Journal of Clinical Psychiatry, 54,* 549–565.

Wallace, J. I., Paauw, D. S., & Spach, D. H. (1993). HIV infection in older patients: When to suspect the unexpected. *Geriatrics, 48,* 61–70.

Wallace, M. (1992). Management of sexual relationships among elderly residents of long term care facilities. *Geriatric Nursing, 13,* 308–311.

Walz, T. H., & Blum, N. S. (1987). *Sexual health in later life.* Lexington, MA: Lexington Books.

Wasow, M., & Loeb, M. B. (1979). Sexuality in nursing homes. *Journal of the American Geriatric Society, 27,* 73–79.

Wasson, J. H., Reda, D. J., Bruskewitz, R. C., Elinson, J., Keller, A. M., & Henderson, W. G. (1995). A comparison of transurethral surgery with watchful waiting for moderate symptoms of benign prostatic hyperplasia. *New England Journal of Medicine, 332,* 75–79.

White, C. B. (1982). A scale for the assessment of attitudes and knowledge regarding sexuality in the aged. *Archives of Sexual Behavior, 11,* 491–502.

White, C. B., & Catania, J. A. (1982). Psychoeducational intervention for sexuality with the aged, family members of the aged, and people who work with the aged. *International Journal of Aging and Human Development, 15,* 121–138.

Wiley, D., & Bortz, W. M. (1996). Sexuality and aging: Usual and successful. *The Journals of Gerontology, 51,* M142–M150.

Williamson, G. M., & Walters, A. S. (1996). Perceived impact of limb amputation on sexual activity: A study of adult amputees. *The Journal of Sex Research, 33,* 221–235.

Winn, R. L., & Newton, N. (1982). Sexuality in aging: A study of 106 cultures. *Archives of Sexual Behavior, 11,* 283–298.

Woessner, J. P. (1963). Age-related changes of the human uterus: Its connective tissue framework. *Journal of Gerontology, 18,* 220–224.

Wolf, D. G. (1982). *Growing older: Lesbians and gay men.* Berkeley: University of California Press.

Zeiss, R. A., Delmonico, R. L., Zeiss, A. M., & Dornbrand, L. (1991). Psychologic disorder and sexual dysfunction in elders. *Clinics in Geriatric Medicine, 7,* 133–151.

Zilbergeld, B. (1992). *The new male sexuality.* New York: Bantam Books.

# Index

An "*f*" or a "*t*" suffix indicates that a term may be found in a figure or table on the page indicated.